Exploring Empathy with Medical Students

David Ian Jeffrey

Exploring Empathy with Medical Students

palgrave
macmillan

David Ian Jeffrey
University of Edinburgh
Edinburgh, UK

ISBN 978-3-030-11210-3 ISBN 978-3-030-11211-0 (eBook)
https://doi.org/10.1007/978-3-030-11211-0

Library of Congress Control Number: 2018966691

This Palgrave Macmillan imprint is published by the registered company Springer Nature Switzerland AG
The registered company address is: Gewerbestrasse 11, 6330 Cham, Switzerland

To Pru

Acknowledgements

I would like to thank the sixteen medical students who took part in this study for sharing their experiences of their undergraduate education, for their enthusiasm and their commitment to the research.

I am grateful to my Ph.D. supervisors, Marilyn Kendall, Marie Fallon, Michael Ross and Lesley Dawson for their patience and wise advice. I owe thanks to Marshall Dozier, Linda Pollock, Scott Murray and many other colleagues who provided helpful advice. I wish to thank Joanna O'Neill, Grace Jackson, Hemapriya Eswanth, Ashwini Elango, Julia Rosche and the publishing team at Palgrave Macmillan for their encouragement and advice.

Thanks also to the Royal College of Physicians of Edinburgh for a Myre Sim bursary to support the costs of transcription of the students' interviews.

Finally, I would like to thank my wife Pru for her support and encouragement.

Contents

1
Introduction

Overview

This chapter outlines the complexity of empathy. It describes the centrality of empathy in patient care and the doctor–patient relationship. The empathy gap in teaching and clinical practice is discussed. The widely reported decline in medical students' empathy is examined. The research approach is described and the audience for the book considered. I describe my motivation for carrying out the study. The chapter concludes with an overview of the book.

The Nature of Empathy

In the scientific literature, empathy is defined in different ways, one definition highlighting the emotional aspect of empathy;

> the natural capacity to share, understand and respond with care to the affective state of others. (Decety 2011, p. vii)

D. I. Jeffrey, *Exploring Empathy with Medical Students*,
https://doi.org/10.1007/978-3-030-11211-0_1

On the other hand, Hojat et al. (2009) take a cognitive view of empathy, excluding emotions but introducing a moral motivation to care.

> Empathy is a predominantly cognitive (as opposed to affective or emotional) attribute that involves an understanding (as opposed to feeling) of patients' experiences, concerns and perspectives, combined with a capacity to communicate this understanding. An intention to help by preventing and alleviating pain and suffering is an additional feature of empathy. (Hojat et al. 2009, p. 1183)

In medical practice and research, empathy is largely viewed as a cognitive construct, leading to a form of professionalism described as 'detached concern' (Hojat et al. 2009; Kelly 2017; Halpern 2001). Alternatively, empathy has been described by combining a number of processes, cognitive, affective, behavioural and moral, in a single concept (Morse et al. 1992). Batson (2011) took yet another view by describing eight different empathies. To add to this conceptual complexity, empathy is often used interchangeably with terms such as compassion and sympathy (Sinclair et al. 2016). Batson (2011) argued that there is a need to clarify the complexity of empathy.

The uncertainty surrounding the definition of empathy has practical implications for research, education and clinical practice (Halpern 2001; Shapiro 2012). Although the various definitions of empathy in the literature share the capacity to understand another person's thoughts and feelings, they differ widely as to whether this capacity includes sharing another's feelings (Decety and Ickes 2011; Batson 2011). The debate surrounding the appropriate emotional content of empathy for clinical practice lies at the heart of this book.

Why Study Empathy?

Empathy enables people to develop and sustain mutually respectful relationships (Cooper 2011). Empathy is an integral part of a trusting patient–doctor relationship (Neumann et al. 2012; Stepien and Baernstein 2006; Derksen et al. 2013; Pedersen 2009). The expression of empathy by healthcare professionals results in improved clinical outcomes and increased patient satisfaction (Derksen et al. 2013; Kim et al. 2004). Pedersen summarised the clinical importance of empathy by explaining that it was needed to understand a patient's illness, their emotional reactions to it and to ascertain what is most important to them, in order to diagnose and treat them appropriately (Pedersen 2010). Empathy also has an ethical role in motivating care and generating altruism (Noddings 1984; Batson et al. 1991).

The General Medical Council (GMC), in defining their outcomes, standards and expectations for undergraduate medical education, highlighted the importance of treating patients as individuals (General Medical Council 2013, 2015). Interest in empathy in medical undergraduate education has increased over the past decades, although most research has been concerned with measuring medical students' empathy rather than seeking to understand the factors which may influence empathy (Underman and Hirshfield 2016; Batt-Rawden et al. 2013; Pedersen 2009).

Despite a general acceptance in the literature of empathy's central role in the patient–doctor relationship, some authors have cautioned that empathy has limits (Macnaughton 2009; Smajdor et al. 2011). They have raised doubts about the extent to which one can understand what another person is thinking and feeling (Macnaughton 2009; Smajdor et al. 2011). However, although it is true that we cannot know completely what it is to think and feel as another person, it is possible to try to imagine the world from the other person's point of view from a basis of our shared humanity. Concerns have been raised in the literature that empathy, in particular its emotional component, might cause burnout in doctors and students, and that emotional empathy might lead to biased clinical judgements (Bloom 2016; Smajdor et al. 2011). This book argues that empathy is integral to medical education and practice and is necessary to provide a balance to mechanistic cognitive-based learning (Cooper 2011).

The Empathy Gap

Although it is accepted that empathy is central to patient care, it is of concern that some high profile reports, such as the Mid Staffordshire NHS Foundation Trust public inquiry, revealed severe failings in patient care (Francis 2010, 2013). The Francis Report identified contributory factors to the gross failures of care; compassion fatigue, overwork, excessive demand, lack of continuity of care and a failure to see the patient as a fellow human being (Haslam 2015; Francis 2013). The Parliamentary Health Service Ombudsman (2011) also found a lack of compassion and a failure to recognise the humanity of frail elderly patients, stating in her report:

> the action of individual staff described here add up to an ignominious failure to look beyond the patient's clinical condition and to respond to the social and emotional needs of the individual and their family. (Parliamentary Health Service Ombudsman 2011, p. 8)

The Parliamentary Health Service Ombudsman concluded that breaches of care were widespread and recommended strongly that the NHS should respond to the failings in care identified in her report (Parliamentary Health Service Ombudsman 2011).

Although the appalling lapses in care described in these reports were not entirely due to a lack of empathy, there is a consensus amongst healthcare professionals that a lack of empathy in the provision of health care in the NHS is a problem (de Zulueta 2013a, b; Cummings and Bennett 2012; Cornwell and Goodrich 2009; Francis 2013; Parliamentary Health Service Ombudsman 2011). Some authors have highlighted the need for doctors to guard against a lack of compassion (Das and Charlton 2018).

Francis (2013) responded to the lack of empathy in patient care by calling for a culture change in the NHS to include more compassionate care. His call for compassion was echoed by the Chief Nursing Officer's recommendation to nurses in the UK (Cummings and Bennett 2012). In a recent report, *Realistic Medicine*, from the Chief Medical Officer, NHS Scotland, Calderwood (2016) highlighted the need for a personalised approach to care and a change to shared decision-making. Berwick (2016) argued for a paradigm change in health care, in the USA, to include listening carefully to the patients' concerns.

The deficit of empathy in clinical practice may in part be due to medicine's dominant biomedical view prioritising technical progress, evidence-based medicine (EBM), targets and efficiency (Shapiro 2012;

de Zulueta 2013a, b; Montgomery 2006). Several authors suggest that healthcare professionals sometimes distance themselves emotionally from patients, by focusing on the biomedical facts, in a process which has been described by Agledahl et al. (2011), as 'existential neglect' or by Halpern (2001), as 'detached concern' (Pedersen 2010; Montgomery 2006).

Some authors point to the context of health care creating a risk of dehumanisation and alienating clinicians from patients (Borgstrom and Walter 2015; de Zulueta 2013a; Zigmond 2011; Haslam 2015). Doctors have complained that their ability to practise empathetically is jeopardised by NHS bureaucracy, causing some patients to feel that their concerns were not addressed adequately (Howick and Rees 2017; Greenhalgh et al. 2014).

Emotions are central to human functioning but academic research in this field is constrained by their complex intangible nature (Cooper 2011). Cooper suggests that emotional empathy reminds us of what medicine is all about (Cooper 2011).

The concerns about a lack of empathy in clinical practice are compounded by a perception, both in medical education research and in society, that medical students' empathy declines during their undergraduate training (Hojat et al. 2009).

A Decline in Medical Students' Empathy

A number of quantitative studies suggest that medical students' empathy declines during their training, particularly during the clinical years of the course (Hojat et al. 2009; Neumann et al. 2011; Pedersen 2009, 2010; Batt-Rawden et al. 2013). However, other researchers have questioned whether this is indeed the case (Quince et al. 2011, 2016b; Colliver et al. 2010; Roff 2015).

The authors of many of the reviews of quantitative studies on students' empathy point out that there is a need to understand the factors which might be influencing the supposed decline in empathy (Pedersen 2010; Batt-Rawden et al. 2013; Quince et al. 2016a; Roff 2015;

Sulzer et al. 2016). They suggest that qualitative research is needed to investigate this problem. The relatively few qualitative studies which have investigated medical students' empathy are mostly cross-sectional rather than longitudinal studies (Tavakol et al. 2012; Lempp and Seale 2004; Eikeland et al. 2014). These qualitative studies identified some factors which enhanced or inhibited empathy but raised further questions as to how empathy changes during undergraduate training and the part played by subtle influences both inside and outside the formal curriculum (Lempp and Seale 2004; Tavakol et al. 2012; Eikeland et al. 2014).

A Phenomenological Approach to Research

Phenomenology is both a philosophy and a research methodology which is concerned with describing the experience of a phenomenon, in this case empathy. This research sought to generate a deeper understanding of medical students' perceptions of empathy and its influences as they progressed through their undergraduate training. The longitudinal qualitative phenomenological study attempted to allow students the space to discuss empathy in a confidential setting. Students could reflect on how they conceptualised empathy in relation to professionalism and practice. They also illustrated influences on their empathy, by describing specific experiences during their undergraduate education. Interviewing students over a three-year period established a foundation of trust between me and student: a relationship which generated a new understanding of empathy and its development in the students' world.

A longitudinal, phenomenological methodology is the most appropriate approach for gaining an understanding of the students' views of empathy and the factors which influence possible changes in their empathy during their training. I imagine phenomenological research as a creative craft like weaving. Developing this simile, the university is the hand-loom, a support structure, with the medical school culture, the vertical warp threads. The students' individual stories become the weft threads which, as a weaver, I select to cross the warp. The differing patterns which emerge from each student's story may be compared to the variety of weaves. The result of my research is not a finished piece of fabric but a sampler. The viewer, or reader, may resonate with some patterns but not others, but each contributes to the sampler and to the debate.

My Motivation to Carry Out the Research

I have been intrigued for many years by how students and doctors resolved the tension between connecting emotionally with patients while maintaining a detached distance from them. As a part of my training in general practice, psychiatry and palliative care, I have been encouraged by role models to share feelings with patients and to be absorbed in exploring the emotional aspects of their illness. I was also interested in the processes of professional and emotional socialisation that students experienced from joining the medical school to graduating as doctors.

I was shocked to read of the appalling lapses in care and lack of empathy outlined in the Francis Report (Francis 2013). I felt that one way of responding to the reported lack of empathy and compassion would be to explore the influences on medical students' empathy during their training, as they are the doctors of the future.

My beliefs at the outset of this project were also informed by quantitative questionnaire-based research, and generally accepted assumptions, which suggested that medical students' empathy declined during their training (Hojat et al. 2009). However, my experience as an academic mentor involved developing close relationships with students which led me to question these assumptions (Jeffrey 2014). I listened as students spoke of their distress at witnessing poor communication with patients, lack of empathy and unethical behaviour by some senior doctors. I therefore wished to explore empathy and the factors influencing any possible change in medical students during their training. I have spent my professional life working with patients in a variety of clinical settings, so I welcomed an opportunity to work in an academic environment, to pause and reflect on my research problem.

Research Aims

The specific aims of this research were to:

1. Explore medical students' conceptualisation of empathy during the undergraduate curriculum.
2. Describe a range of students' views and experiences of factors influencing their empathy during their training.
3. Synthesise and interpret the findings to gain understanding of how and why medical students' empathy changes during their training.
4. Consider how this understanding might inform medical undergraduate training and improve patient care in the future.

Audience for the Book

Medical educators and those involved with undergraduate education may engage with the findings of this research. The insights gained from this work may also resonate with those involved in postgraduate medical training. Although the study is focused on empathy in medical students, the literature draws from research in nursing, counselling, social work and from the training of allied healthcare professionals, so may be of interest to these professionals and their teachers. The General Medical Council (GMC) may be informed by this research in their approaches to patient-centred care, professionalism and undergraduate medical education.

Medical students may find this research of interest in their professional development in becoming both competent and caring doctors. Empathy affects all human relationships so this research in a wider sense may be of interest to policy-makers, patients and the public, who want to gain a deeper understanding of the medical students who will be their doctors in future.

The nature of this phenomenological study is to present findings which encourage debate. My conclusions are necessarily tentative but may resonate with the reader, and be transferable to other medical schools, contributing to the promotion of empathy in curriculum development and patient care.

Overview of the Book

Chapter 1: Introduction

This chapter outlines the complexity of empathy. It describes the centrality of empathy in patient care and the doctor–patient relationship. The empathy gap in teaching and clinical practice is discussed. The widely reported decline in medical students' empathy is examined. The research approach is described and the audience for the book considered. I describe my motivation for carrying out the study. The chapter concludes with an overview of the book.

Chapter 2: The Research Setting and Study Design

In this chapter, I briefly justify the choice of a phenomenological approach to explore the students' views and to gain new understanding about empathy. I outline the medical school setting and curriculum, the participants, the study design and describe interpretative phenomenological analysis as the approach to data analysis.

Chapter 3: Empathy: From Attribute to Relationship

This chapter discusses the change in students' perceptions of empathy as they gain clinical experience with patients. Initially they talk about as empathy as a possession, something that they have. Later, they see empathy as something that they do, as a dynamic process which is embedded in a relationship and much affected by the context of the clinical consultation with the patient.

Chapter 4: Emotions and Empathy: Risks and Benefits of Emotional Connection with a Patient

Students describe the risks and benefits of emotional connection with a patient. They describe how they are taught to distance themselves from patients and so come to see this as being 'professional'. The model for detached concern in professionalism is described and explored. They discuss ways in which they strike a balance between connection and attachment. Appropriate boundary setting is explored.

Chapter 5: Enhancing Empathy
In this chapter, the students identify the factors which encourage empathy with patients. The main factor is their contact with patients, supported by an experienced clinician. They describe aspects of teaching and support which they found helpful.

Chapter 6: Barriers to Empathy: The Medical School Culture
This chapter addresses the hidden curriculum, the culture, or ambience, of the medical school. The medical school studied is rated highly for research but receives low ratings from students for their teaching experience. In this chapter, many aspects of the hidden curriculum are made explicit. The links between student well-being, stress and empathy are discussed.

Chapter 7: Barriers to Empathy: The Curriculum
This chapter addresses the formal curriculum and its effects on empathy. The chapter begins with a discussion of whether empathy can be taught. The students describe a lack of teaching about empathy and the neglect of psychosocial aspects of the patient's situation. They talk about the strong biomedical bias in their teaching and its negative effect of empathy. Other barriers such as negative role models, assessment and feedback are explored in relation to the student–patient relationship.

Chapter 8: Changes in Students' Empathy During Their Training
A widely accepted view that students' empathy declines during their training is contested by the experience of the students in this study. Instead, they describe an increasing focus on the patient, distress at examples of a lack of empathy with patients and a concern that they remain empathetic doctors in the future. They also describe the ways in which in some clinical situations they hide expression of their empathy in the interests of appearing 'efficient'.

Chapter 9: Summary and Implications
This chapter summarises the key findings of this innovative research. I hope these conclusions will resonate with medical educators who may appreciate the insights gained from the students' stories. In any

phenomenological research, drawing implications for undergraduate medical education must be tentative. Implications for the medical school culture and for the curriculum are debated.

Key Points

This research sought to answer the following questions:

- How do students talk about and experience the concept of empathy in relation to professionalism and practice?
- What factors do medical students describe as influencing their empathy during their undergraduate medical training?
- How do medical students' views and experiences of empathy change during their medical education?

References

Agledahl, K. M., Gulbrandsen, P., Førde, R., & Wifstad, Å. (2011). Courteous but not curious: How doctors' politeness masks their existential neglect—A qualitative study of video-recorded patient consultations. *Journal of Medical Ethics, 37,* 650–654.

Batson, C. (2011). These things called empathy: Eight related but distinct phenomena. In J. Decety & W. Ickes (Eds.), *The Social Neuroscience of Empathy.* Cambridge: MIT Press.

Batson, C. D., Batson, J. G., Slingsby, J., Harrell, K. L., Peekna, H. M., & Todd, R. M. (1991). Empathic joy and the empathy-altruism hypothesis. *Journal of Personality and Social Psychology, 61,* 413–426.

Batt-Rawden, S., Chisolm, M. S., Anton, B., & Flickinger, T. E. (2013). Teaching empathy to medical students: An updated, systematic review. *Academic Medicine, 88,* 1171–1177.

Berwick, D. M. (2016). Era 3 for medicine and health care. *JAMA, 315,* 1329–1330.

Bloom, P. (2016). *Against Empathy: The Case for Rational Compassion.* London: The Bodley Head.

Borgstrom, E., & Walter, T. (2015). Choice and compassion at the end of life: A critical analysis of recent English policy discourse. *Social Science and Medicine, 136,* 99–105.

Calderwood, C. (2016). *Realistic Medicine: Chief Medical Officer's Annual Report 2014–2015.* Edinburgh: Scottish Government.

Colliver, J. A., Conlee, M., Verhulst, S. J., & Dorsey, J. K. (2010). Reports of the decline of empathy during medical education are greatly exaggerated: A re-examination of the research. *Academic Medicine, 85,* 588–593.

Cooper, B. (2011). *Empathy in Education: Engagement, Values and Achievement.* London: Bloomsbury Publishing.

Cornwell, J., & Goodrich, J. (2009). Exploring how to enable compassionate care in hospital to improve patient experience. *Nursing Times, 105,* 14–21.

Cummings, J., & Bennett, V. (2012). *Compassion in Practice: Nursing, Midwifery and Care Staff: Our Vision and Strategy.* London: NHS England.

Das, A., & Charlton, R. (2018). Guarding against dispassion for doctors in the NHS. *Journal of the Royal Society of Medicine, 111*(10), 359–365.

de Zulueta, P. (2013a). Compassion in 21st century medicine: Is it sustainable? *Clinical Ethics, 8,* 119–128.

de Zulueta, P. (2013b). Responding to the Francis report some simple but radical suggestions. *Journal of Holistic Healthcare, 10*(1), 20–22.

Decety, J. (2011). *Empathy: From Bench to Bedside.* Cambridge: MIT Press.

Decety, J., & Ickes, W. (2011). *The Social Neuroscience of Empathy.* Cambridge: MIT Press.

Derksen, F., Bensing, J., & Lagro-Janssen, A. (2013). Effectiveness of empathy in general practice: A systematic review. *British Journal General Practice, 63*(606), 76–84.

Eikeland, H. L., Ornes, K., Finset, A., & Pedersen, R. (2014). The physician's role and empathy—A qualitative study of third year medical students. *BMC Medical Education, 14*(1), 165–173.

Francis, R. (2010). *The Independent Inquiry into Care Provided by Mid-Staffordshire NHS Foundation Trust, January 2005–March 2009.* London: HMSO.

Francis, R. (2013). *Report of the Mid Staffordshire NHS Foundation Trust Public Inquiry: Executive Summary.* London: HMSO.

General Medical Council. (2013). *Good Medical Practice.* London: General Medical Council.

General Medical Council. (2015). *Outcomes for Graduates (Tomorrow's Doctors).* London: General Medical Council.

Greenhalgh, T., Howick, J., & Maskrey, N. (2014). Evidence based medicine: A movement in crisis? *British Medical Journal, 348,* g3725.
Halpern, J. (2001). *From Detached Concern to Empathy: Humanizing Medical Practice.* Oxford: Oxford University Press.
Haslam, D. (2015). More than kindness. *Journal of Compassionate Health Care, 2,* 6–9.
Hojat, M., Vergare, M. J., Maxwell, K., Brainard, G., Herrine, S. K., Isenberg, G. A., et al. (2009). The devil is in the third year: A longitudinal study of erosion of empathy in medical school. *Academic Medicine, 84*(9), 1182–1191.
Howick, J., & Rees, S. (2017). Overthrowing barriers to empathy in healthcare: Empathy in the age of the internet. *Journal of the Royal Society of Medicine, 110*(9), 1–6.
Jeffrey, D. (2014). *Medical Mentoring: Supporting Students, Doctors in Training and General Practitioners.* London: Royal College of General Practitioners.
Kelly, J. (2017). When I say…empathy. *Medical Education, 51*(6), 573–574.
Kim, S. S., Kaplowitz, S., & Johnston, M. V. (2004). The effects of physician empathy on patient satisfaction and compliance. *Evaluation and the Health Professions, 27*(3), 237–251.
Lempp, H., & Seale, C. (2004). The hidden curriculum in undergraduate medical education: Qualitative study of medical students' perceptions of teaching. *British Medical Journal, 329,* 770–773.
Macnaughton, J. (2009). The dangerous practice of empathy. *Lancet, 373,* 1940–1941.
Montgomery, K. (2006). *How Doctors Think: Clinical Judgment and the Practice of Medicine.* Oxford: Oxford University Press.
Morse, J. M., Anderson, G., Bottorff, J. L., Yonge, O., O'Brien, B., Solberg, S., et al. (1992). Exploring empathy: A conceptual fit for nursing practice? *Image: The Journal of Nursing Scholarship, 24*(4), 273–280.
Neumann, M., Edelhaeuser, F., Tauschel, D., Fischer, M. R., Wirtz, M., Woopen, C., et al. (2011). Empathy decline and its reasons: A systematic review of studies with medical students and residents. *Academic Medicine, 86*(8), 996–1009.
Neumann, M., Scheffer, C., Tauschel, D., Lutz, G., Wirtz, M., & Edelhauser, F. (2012). Physician empathy: Definition, outcome-relevance and its measurement in patient care and medical education. *GMS Zeitschrift fur medizinische Ausbildung, 29*(1), 1–21.

Noddings, N. (1984). *Caring: A Feminine Approach to Ethics and Moral Education*. Berkeley: University of California Press.
Parliamentary Health Service Ombudsman. (2011). *Care and Compassion? Report of the Health Service Ombudsman on Ten Investigations into NHS Care of Older People*. London: HMSO.
Pedersen, R. (2009). Empirical research on empathy in medicine—A critical review. *Patient Education and Counseling, 76*(3), 307–322.
Pedersen, R. (2010). Empathy development in medical education—A critical review. *Medical Teacher, 32*(7), 593–600.
Quince, T. A., Parker, R. A., Wood, D., & Benson, J. A. (2011). Stability of empathy among undergraduate medical students: A longitudinal study at one UK medical school. *BMC Medical Education, 11*(1), 90–99.
Quince, T., Thiemann, P., Benson, J., & Hyde, S. (2016a). Undergraduate medical students' empathy: Current perspectives. *Advances in Medical Education and Practice, 7*, 443–455.
Quince, T. A., Kinnersley, P., Hales, J., da Silva, A., Moriarty, H., Thiemann, P., et al. (2016b). Empathy among undergraduate medical students: A multi-centre cross-sectional comparison of students beginning and approaching the end of their course. *BMC Medical Education, 16*, 92–102.
Roff, S. (2015). Reconsidering the "decline" of medical student empathy as reported in studies using the Jefferson scale of physician empathy-student version (JSPE-S). *Medical Teacher, 37*(8), 783–786.
Shapiro, J. (2012). The paradox of teaching empathy in medical students. In J. Decety (Ed.), *Empathy: From Bench to Bedside*. Cambridge: MIT Press.
Sinclair, S., Norris, J. M., McConnell, S. J., Chochinov, H. M., Hack, T., Hagen, N. A., et al. (2016). Compassion: A scoping review of the health-care literature. *BMC Palliative Care, 15*, 6–22.
Smajdor, A., Stöckl, A., & Salter, C. (2011). The limits of empathy: Problems in medical education and practice. *Journal of Medical Ethics, 37*(6), 380–383.
Stepien, K. A., & Baernstein, A. (2006). Educating for empathy—A review. *Journal of General Internal Medicine, 21*(5), 524–530.
Sulzer, S. H., Feinstein, N. W., & Wendland, C. L. (2016). Assessing empathy development in medical education: A systematic review. *Medical Education, 50*(3), 300–310.

Tavakol, S., Dennick, R., & Tavakol, M. (2012). Medical students' understanding of empathy: A phenomenological study. *Medical Education, 46*(3), 306–316.
Underman, K., & Hirshfield, L. E. (2016). Detached concern? Emotional socialization in twenty-first century medical education. *Social Science and Medicine, 160,* 94–101.
Zigmond, D. (2011). Five executive follies: How commodification imperils compassion in person healthcare. *Journal Holistic Healthcare, 9,* 7–10.

2
The Research Setting and Study Design

Overview

In this chapter, the theoretical framework of the research, phenomenology and interpretative phenomenological analysis (IPA) as the approach to data analysis are described. The medical school, the research setting and the curriculum are defined. The process of the research, the study design, is discussed.

Theoretical Framework

Qualitative research is based on subjectivity and is concerned with how the social world is interpreted, experienced and understood (Cleland 2015). Most research into empathy in medical students has been quantitative in design and grounded in a realist ontology. Realism maintains that objective knowledge from hypothesis generation, e.g. a decline in students' empathy during training, can be discovered by scientific investigation using positivist methods, e.g. a questionnaire survey and statistical analysis. However, I was interested in exploring and understanding

D. I. Jeffrey, *Exploring Empathy with Medical Students*,
https://doi.org/10.1007/978-3-030-11211-0_2

the meaning of the students' experiences and views on empathy. I have therefore adopted a relativist ontology which accepts that the representation of things in the world is socially constructed and cannot be taken as a simple reflection of how things are (Mann and MacLeod 2015). My constructivist epistemology proposes that knowledge is gained through subjective understanding and interpretations (Crotty 1998; Mann and MacLeod 2015). Constructivism is concerned with making sense of the lived world, in my research, from the standpoint of the student (Mann 2011). It maintains that meanings do not exist in some external world but are created by the subject's interaction with the world. As a result, multiple constructed accounts of the world can exist (Crotty 1998). I sought to understand how the students interacted with patients, their peers and teachers in a variety of settings. I then explored how these interactions changed during their course.

Phenomenology

Phenomenology is a term which describes both a philosophy and a range of research approaches (Finlay 2013). Phenomenology aims at gaining a deeper understanding of the meaning of our everyday, taken for granted, experiences as they are lived (Van Manen 2016, p. 9). It can also be described as a way of seeing how things appear to us through experience, from an individual's perspective (Finlay 2013; Carel 2016; Smith et al. 2009). Using a phenomenological method, I sought to understand the individual student's perspective of their education (Hopkins et al. 2017). Phenomenology focuses on phenomena (what we perceive and experience) rather than the reality of things (what there is) (Carel 2016). It asserts that any effort to understand the students' world has to be grounded in their experience of their social reality (Crotty 1998).

This qualitative research aimed to develop an interpreted understanding of the students' social world focused on their everyday experience in relation to empathy (McMillan 2015; McLeod 2011; Kvale and Brinkmann 2009). Although interpretative research may not generate neat parcels of knowledge, it can provide insights into the students' social world. A longitudinal phenomenological approach allowed the students' stories to develop and was a more appropriate methodology to capture change than the static 'snapshot' gained in cross-sectional research. Qualitative longitudinal research (QLR) has been underused in previous studies of empathy in medical students, perhaps because it is more challenging to carry out than a cross-sectional study (Murray et al. 2009; Pedersen 2009). A QLR methodology was more likely to reveal a nuanced in-depth understanding of empathy since it provided an opportunity for strengthening my relationship with the student, fostered trust, and gave students the chance to clarify or change their views (McLeod 2011; Holland et al. 2006). The research also interrogated the data across time, both in the individual student's story and in relation to the larger group in each year (Holland et al. 2006). This approach offered the best chance of gaining a coherent, nuanced understanding of the individual student and of the group of students in context.

Finlay (2008) described the phenomenological attitude as a reductive–reflexive dance where the researcher adopts two stances between bracketing pre-understandings and exploiting them as a source of insight (Finlay 2008). Therefore, the reader and I bring our assumptions to the book and cannot help but look at any new text in the light of our own prior experience (Smith et al. 2009). The description of the research method may give an impression of a linear progression of steps when in fact this circular process is a truer reflection of the interpretation. The research involved a double hermeneutic: my interpretation of the student's interpretation their experience. Indeed, when the reader interprets my research a third hermeneutic level exists. Halling (2007) suggests that phenomenological research involves three levels of data analysis: the individual student's experience, common themes amongst the students and finally a more abstract philosophical reflection on the nature of empathy.

Interpretative Phenomenological Analysis (IPA)

Interpretative phenomenological analysis (IPA) was developed in the 1990s and has mostly been used in psychology and nursing research, but only rarely in medical education research (Smith et al. 2009).

As Larkin et al. (2006) point out, the analytic processes of IPA shares common features with other qualitative methods and so it is more appropriate to understand IPA as a stance from which to approach the qualitative data analysis rather than a distinct method (Larkin et al. 2006). Critics of the phenomenological approach often argue against its relativism (Paley 2017). However, a phenomenological approach is not a matter of 'anything goes', but rather an acknowledgement that different people perceive differently and act differently. I hope the reader will also examine the stories from the perspective of their own experiential knowledge base, make their interpretations and consider possible implications for further work.

The Process of the Research

Any understanding from research, informs the reader both about the students' views of empathy and about my own suppositions. Heidegger maintained that interpretation was an inevitable basic structure of our 'being in' the world (Heidegger 1962/1927). The interpretative revelation of the phenomenon, empathy, and the reflexive uncovering of the self are integral parts of the same process (Finlay and Gough 2008). I used reflexivity throughout the research when considering; my motivation, 'bracketing' and the researcher–student relationship. It was also involved in data generation, analysis and in the assurance of the quality of the research.

The Study Design

The study employed a prospective qualitative longitudinal phenomenological methodology. A purposive sample of two cohorts of eight medical students was followed for three academic years of their undergraduate training, thus covering the entire curriculum. The cohorts fell into two groups:

- Preclinical Group: (8 students) Five students were followed from year 1 to year 3. Three students opted not to undertake the intercalated science year (year 3) and their data for year 4 was included in the Clinical Group.
- Clinical Group: (8 students) Eight students were followed from years 3 to year 6. Three students from the Preclinical Group entered year 4 and their data for this year was included in the Clinical Group.

Data was generated using in-depth, one-to-one interviews of students. Interviews with students were carried out in an office on the medical school premises and lasted 60–90 minutes. Interviews were audio-recorded and transcribed by an experienced medical administrator.

Ethical Perspectives

I ensured that the students volunteered and understood the meaning of the study. Their stories were not distorted, their anonymity was protected and their welfare was my primary concern (Karnieli-Miller et al. 2009). Informed consent was a process which pervaded the whole research process. Each student signed a consent form which was reviewed before every interview.

Formal ethical approvals for the study were obtained from the Centre for Population Health Sciences (CPHS) Level 2 Ethics Committee and the College of Medicine and Veterinary Medicine Students' Ethics Committee (MVMSEC).

The need for anonymity and confidentiality of students potentially clashed with placing their accounts in the public arena. I decided that I would provide minimal information about the background of the students, by giving them a pseudonym, guaranteeing their anonymity. I did not overtly identify the medical school where the studied was carried out. Interview transcripts were held on the university password protected server in accordance with Data Protection Act and the university regulations (Holland et al. 2006).

Research Setting: The Medical School

The students attended a UK medical school which has an outstanding record in medical research but has low student ratings for teaching and student experience (National Student Survey 2017). The stated aim of their undergraduate programme is to produce caring, competent, ethical and reflective doctors who make care of patients their first concern. The programme overview of the medical school lists the following distinctive features of the educational experience at this medical school including:

- An emphasis on the sciences and humanities underpinning clinical practice.
- Research skills and enquiry-led learning.
- A blend of traditional and innovative teaching and learning methods that includes lectures, problem-based learning, e-learning, simulation workshops, portfolio learning and clinical attachments.
- A personal tutor system to ensure students are well supported in their academic and professional development and know how to access pastoral support and career guidance.

The Medical Undergraduate Curriculum

The curriculum structure is summarised in Table 2.1. In the preclinical years from 1 to 3, there is only a limited patient contact. In years 4–6, the curriculum takes students through the major systems-based clinical specialities in hospital and community-based attachments. By Year 6, students are regarded as ready to learn and contribute to the care of patients as apprentices under careful supervision.

In addition to the timetable, the curriculum can be described in terms of the intended learning outcomes of each part of the course. The medical degree (MBChB) outcome is defined through twelve programme learning outcomes each of which is addressed in every year of the course. The twelve outcomes are subdivided into: The Doctor as

Table 2.1 The medical curriculum

Year 1	Principles of practice	**Preclinical**: Cardiovascular, Respiratory, Locomotor Health ethics and society; Problem-based learning Year 1 Theme teaching
2	Principles of practice	**Preclinical**: Neurosciences, Gastrointestinal, Genetics < renal endocrine and the virtual clinic Introduction to clinical practice, Problem-based learning Year 2 Theme teaching
3	Intercalated bachelor of medical sciences (honours)	**Preclinical**: Science honours degree
4	Process of care	**Clinical**: Cardiovascular, Respiratory, Locomotor, Gastrointestinal, Psychiatry Year 4 Theme teaching
5	Process of care	**Clinical**: Haematology, Oncology, Renal, Neurosciences, Dermatology, Ophthalmology, Otolaryngology, General practice, Obstetrics and Gynaecology, Genitourinary medicine, Psychiatry Year 5 Theme teaching
6	Preparation for professional practice	**Clinical**: Child life and health, Medicine, General practice, Medicine of elderly, Surgery Student assistantship and elective Year 6 Theme teaching

a Scholar and Scientist (4), The Doctor as a Practitioner (6) and The Doctor as a Professional (2) (General Medical Council 2015).

The medical school does not conduct selection interviews. The words 'empathy' or 'compassion' do not appear anywhere in the document describing the medical degree programme (MBChB) at this university. A recent curriculum change made the intercalated science honours degree compulsory, increasing duration of the curriculum to six years. The brief map of the curriculum describes the context of the medical undergraduate course but the students' accounts provide a richer view of their perceptions of their teaching (Table 2.1).

Sixteen Medical Students

The sampling of medical students was purposive and consistent with my phenomenological approach. I recruited on the basis of first-come-first-included as I wished to represent perspectives rather than a population (Silverman 2013). This number of students allowed me to retain a close trusting relationship with each of them which was necessary to generate rich data (Flyvbjerg 2006; McMillan 2015).

Eight first-year students (6 females and 2 males) and eight fourth-year students (7 females and 1 male) consented to join the study. Although I was not making any claim that the group was representative of the whole year groups, I was pleased to have recruited a diverse group of three males and thirteen female students. The first-year students in the preclinical group included an overseas graduate student, a British Asian and a student from Europe, the remainder were school-leavers from the UK. With the exception of the graduate student, the school-leavers had attended care homes or GP surgeries for up to two weeks before joining university to gain experience. The fourth-year students, in the clinical group, included one student who had completed their preclinical studies at another university. One student was Chinese, one a British Asian, one was from a European country and the remainder were UK-based students. Six students in the clinical group had undertaken an intercalated honours science year. I assigned a pseudonym for each student.

Data Generation

Data were generated by using semi-structured interviews which developed into student-led conversations as study progressed. Interviews remain the best source of knowledge about the students' feelings (Hitchings 2012). I was present in the interview as a witness rather than an authority. Kvale and Brinkmann (2009) asserted that our understanding of other people's lived experience depended on conversation, reflecting Gadamer's views of the role of conversation in generating meaning (Gadamer 1990/1960).

Transcribing

The transcribing was carried out by an experienced medical administrator. To elucidate the meaning and increase readability, I have edited the quotes from the students' transcripts in the thesis only to remove repetitions, e.g. 'and', 'erm', 'um', 'like', 'so', 'you know' and other mannerisms of speech, which might have made the student identifiable to their colleagues. I use an ellipsis [...] in the quotes to indicate where text has been omitted. I have not corrected the grammatical errors in the quotes.

Interpretative Phenomenological Analysis (IPA) (Figure 2.1)

Although my description listed a number of steps, in practice the analytic process was iterative, going back and forth from the data to my analysis and from the particular to the general. The iterative process is described in detail in a number of steps which are summarised in Fig. 2.1 (Smith et al. 2009):

1. I began by listening to the recording of each student's interview and correcting any 'typos' in the transcript.
2. I re-read the transcripts, immersing myself in the content and making rough notes of important themes that emerged from the data (Saldana 2013).
3. I downloaded the transcript on NVivo 10, a computer software programme, that I used to store the data and for my coding (Bazeley and Jackson 2013).
4. I carried out a close reading of the transcript, line by line, analysing the claims, concerns and understandings of the student. In doing so, I identified emergent themes, commonalities and divergences (Saldana 2013).
5. For each theme, I created a keyword or code on NVivo 10 and stored the relevant part of the transcript within the code (Saldana 2013).

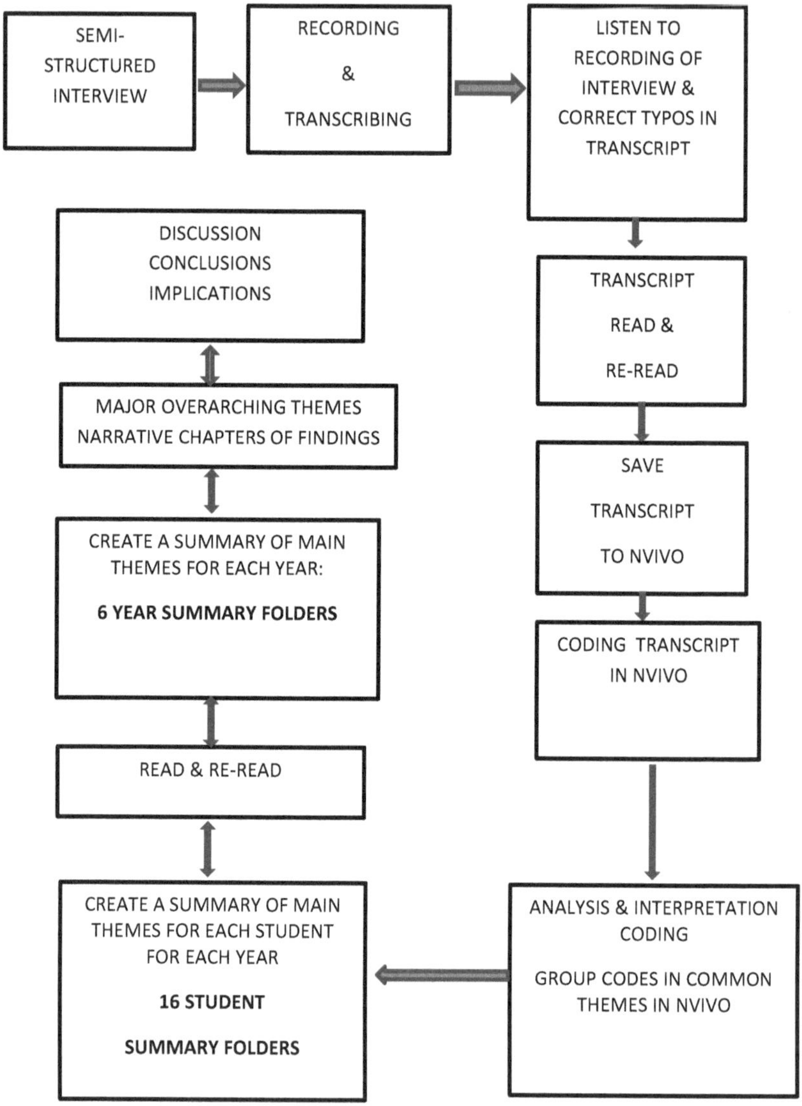

Fig. 2.1 Data analysis using interpretative phenomenological analysis

6. As the themes developed in the story, I found that some parts could be coded within a number of themes. I wrote memos to remind myself of how the codes had developed recorded ideas about

my interpretation and listed questions to follow up in the next interview.

7. A framework of codes was derived from the data. It was important to my phenomenological approach that the coding framework emerged from the reading and re-reading of the transcripts and was not imposed on the data (Smith et al. 2009).
8. After each student's transcript had been coded, I wrote an individual interpretative summary of their story and the themes that had emerged.
9. Once I had completed a student's story, I moved to analyse another student's story in the same year of their study.
10. I repeated the analysis for each student year by year and completed an individual folder for each student with three years of my summarised data analysis. I read and re-read these folders to become familiar with the data and my interpretations.
11. After completing the analysis of eight transcripts in each year of the course, I looked at the themes across each year in turn. I wrote a summary of my interpretation of the views of the students in each year of the course, developing six folders, with an analysis for each year. This iterative process involved comparing not just the individual from one interview to the next but also looking across each year in a cross-sectional way to gain understandings from the whole group.
12. Themes emerged as the data were scrutinised, generating new insights. Analysis was an iterative process with emergent themes informing future interviews. As this was a longitudinal data analysis it also focused on how the student' views changed over time (Murray et al. 2009).
13. Reflection of my perception and process led to a more interpretative approach involving the hermeneutic circle of moving between the part and the whole. In this way, a framework evolved which illustrated the relationship between themes. My coding frameworks, notes and supervision reports form an audit trail of this analytic process.
14. This process led to the development of a full narrative detailing the connections theme by theme. My constructivist epistemology

acknowledged that the interpretations I offered were tentative and that other researchers might interpret the data in a different way.
15. Finally, a full narrative was developed with a commentary on the data generated which takes the reader through the interpretation theme by theme.

The process of analysis is set out in Fig. 2.1.

Quality of the Research

The consolidated criteria for reporting qualitative research (COREQ) were used as checklist that ensured that the most important aspects of the study methods were reported (Tong et al. 2007). Qualitative methods share an interest in analysing data to explore meaning rather than statistical differences or relationships. Notions of trustworthiness, strength and transferability of knowledge in social sciences are equivalent to reliability, validity and generalization in quantitative research (Kvale and Brinkmann 2009). Validity of qualitative research is concerned with whether my interpretations fit the description of the account. As there is no single correct interpretation the reader has to ask, 'Is the explanation credible'? The concept of reliability is replaced in this research by the notion of trustworthiness of the researcher. As phenomenological–interpretative research is at its heart a creative endeavour, there was a need to follow one's intuition and not to stifle creativity (Kvale and Brinkmann 2009). My transcripts, student summary folders and year summary folders, notes, supervision meetings, and my reflexivity formed an audit trail and demonstrated my commitment, rigour and sensitivity to the research.

Kvale proposed the concept of craftsmanship rather than validity in qualitative research (Kvale and Brinkmann 2009). Craftsmanship involves the credibility of researcher, the questioning of findings and their interpretation. I have adopted this model of craftsmanship from the outset of my research by relating my phenomenological investigation with weaving. Rather than generalising from my research, I sought to explore to the extent to which the findings at one medical school were transferrable to other institutions and students. Conclusions from interpretative-phenomenological research are necessarily tentative but I hope that the insights presented in this thesis resonate with my readers and particularly with those involved in medical education.

Key Points

- A qualitative approach is appropriate to gain an understanding of the students' views of empathy.
- Phenomenology aims to gain a deeper understanding of the meaning of our experiences.
- A longitudinal approach allowed the students' stories to develop and to capture change.

The students claimed that the medical school has an emphasis on biomedical science.

References

Bazeley, P., & Jackson, K. (2013). *Qualitative Data Analysis with NVIVO*. London: Sage.

Carel, H. (2016). *The Phenomenology of Illness*. Oxford: Oxford University Press.

Cleland, J. (2015). Exploring versus measuring: Considering the fundamental differences between qualitative and quantitative research. In J. Cleland & S. Durning (Eds.), *Researching Medical Education*. London: Wiley.

Crotty, M. (1998). *The Foundations of Social Research: Meaning and Perspective in the Research Process*. London: Sage.

Finlay, L. (2008). A dance between the reduction and reflexivity: Explicating the "phenomenological psychological attitude". *Journal of Phenomenological Psychology, 39*, 1–32.

Finlay, L. (2013). Unfolding the phenomenological research process: Iterative stages of "seeing afresh". *Journal of Humanistic Psychology, 53*, 172–201.

Finlay, L., & Gough, B. (2008). *Reflexivity: A Practical Guide for Researchers in Health and Social Sciences*. Chichester: Wiley.

Flyvbjerg, B. (2006). Five misunderstandings about case-study research. *Qualitative Inquiry, 12,* 219–245.
Gadamer, H. (1990/1960). *Truth and Method.* New York: Crossroad.
General Medical Council. (2015). *Outcomes for Graduates (Tomorrow's Doctors).* London: General Medical Council.
Halling, S. (2007). *Intimacy, Transcendence, and Psychology: Closeness and Openness in Everyday Life.* Basingstoke: Palgrave Macmillan.
Heidegger, M. (1962/1927). *Being and Time.* Oxford: Blackwell.
Hitchings, R. (2012). People can talk about their practices. *Area, 44,* 61–67.
Holland, J., Thomson, R., & Henderson, S. (2006). *Qualitative Longitudinal Research: A Discussion Paper.* London: South Bank University.
Hopkins, R. M., Regehr, G., & Pratt, D. D. (2017). A framework for negotiating positionality in phenomenological research. *Medical Teacher, 39,* 20–25.
Karnieli-Miller, O., Strier, R., & Pessach, L. (2009). Power relations in qualitative research. *Qualitative Health Research, 19,* 279–289.
Kvale, S., & Brinkmann, S. (2009). *Interviews: Learning the Craft of Qualitative Research Interviewing.* London: Sage.
Larkin, M., Watts, S., & Clifton, E. (2006). Giving voice and making sense in interpretative phenomenological analysis. *Qualitative Research in Psychology, 3,* 102–120.
Mann, K. V. (2011). Theoretical perspectives in medical education: Past experience and future possibilities. *Medical Education, 45,* 60–68.
Mann, K., & MacLeod, A. (2015). Constructivism: Learning theories and approaches to research. In J. Cleland & S. Durning (Eds.), *Researching Medical Education.* London: Wiley.
McLeod, J. (2011). *Qualitative Research in Counselling and Psychotherapy.* London: Sage.
McMillan, W. (2015). Theory in healthcare education research: The importance of worldview. In J. Cleland & S. Durning (Eds.), *Researching Medical Education.* London: Wiley.
Murray, S. A., Kendall, M., Carduff, E., Worth, A., Harris, F. M., Lloyd, A., et al. (2009). Use of serial qualitative interviews to understand patients' evolving experiences and needs. *BMJ, 339,* b3702.
National Student Survey. (2017). *Times Higher Education Supplement* [Online]. Available https://www.timeshighereducation.com/student/news/national-student-survey-2017-overall-satisfaction-results. Accessed December 27, 2017.

Paley, J. (2017). *Phenomenology as Qualitative Research: A Critical Analysis of Meaning Attribution*. London: Taylor & Francis.

Pedersen, R. (2009). Empirical research on empathy in medicine—A critical review. *Patient Education and Counseling, 76*, 307–322.

Saldana, J. (2013). *The Coding Manual for Qualitative Researchers*. London: Sage.

Silverman, D. (2013). *Doing Qualitative Research: A Practical Handbook*. London: Sage.

Smith, J. A., Flowers, P., & Larkin, M. (2009). *Interpretative Phenomenological Analysis: Theory, Method and Research*. London: Sage.

Tong, A., Sainsbury, P., & Craig, J. (2007). Consolidated criteria for reporting qualitative research (COREQ): A 32-item checklist for interviews and focus groups. *International Journal for Quality in Health Care, 19*, 349–357.

Van Manen, M. (2016). *Researching Lived Experience: Human Science for an Action Sensitive Pedagogy*. London: Routledge.

3
Empathy: From Attribute to Relationship

Overview

The importance of empathy and the way the construct has evolved are discussed. Initially, students described empathy as a personal attribute, but in the clinical years they changed their view describing empathy as a relational construct dependent upon the context of the meeting with a patient. The students reflected on the process of empathising.

The Significance of Empathy

Students saw empathy as part of a trusting patient–doctor relationship which resulted in improved health outcomes and increased satisfaction for patients. They suggested that empathising enabled a patient to voice their real concerns and so to be more involved in their care.

> if you feel that your doctor understands you then you are more inclined to talk about mental health issues, social issues. (Edward, Year 1)

D. I. Jeffrey, *Exploring Empathy with Medical Students*,
https://doi.org/10.1007/978-3-030-11211-0_3

Some students described empathy as a bridge equalising power between a doctor and a patient. This empathetic connection ensured that treatment decisions met the patient's goals of care. Helen noticed that some patients in a chemotherapy clinic seemed to agree to the doctor's treatment plan without questioning.

> quite often patients[are] just going through with treatment just because it is what you do. (Helen, Year 1)

Some students claimed that empathy enabled the patient to feel acknowledged as a human being, not merely as an object of scientific interest, so differentiating medicine from a technical job. Others asserted that empathy was a fundamental virtue of being a doctor.

> I think that if you don't have any empathy then you see the patient as an object. What defines, well makes, medicine different from say being a mechanic. (Lisa, Year 4)

Pedersen emphasised the centrality of empathy to patient care;

> Empathic understanding is needed not only to understand the patient's illness or emotional reactions but also to understand adequately what is at stake for the patient and to diagnose and treat the patient adequately, to avoid acting against the patient's will, and to throw into relief the patient's and the physician's horizon. Furthermore, keeping empathic understanding separate from the natural scientific aspects of medicine helps to sustain a stubborn misconception; that is, empathic understanding is radically different from other aspects of clinical understanding. (Pedersen 2010, p. 597).

There are many factors which contribute to a patient's clinical outcome, making it difficult to identify the impact of empathy. Historically, the patient–doctor relationship has been regarded as having important therapeutic effects (Balint 1957; Di Blasi et al. 2001). Recent systematic reviews have confirmed that the quality of the patient–doctor relationship had a small but significant effect on patient health outcomes (Kelley et al. 2014; Howick et al. 2018b). Patients have described how much they desired empathetic care (Broyard 1992; Little et al. 2001; Coulter 2002; Wensing et al. 1998; Derksen et al. 2013).

Some research suggests that empathy can improve health outcomes, for example, in certain patients with diabetes, pain and even the common cold (Hojat et al. 2011; Del Canale et al. 2012; Rakel et al. 2009; Neumann et al. 2007; Price et al. 2006). Perhaps the best understood process by which empathy improves health outcomes lies in the patient's perception of the doctor's concern and trust (Halpern 2012; Ballatt and Campling 2011). The General Medical Council (GMC) emphasises the importance of trust and describes compassion as a professional skill that makes a good doctor (General Medical Council 2009, 2013, 2015). In a trusting empathetic relationship, patients may disclose more of their symptoms and concerns, leading to a more accurate diagnosis and to patients feeling involved in their care (Roter et al. 1998; Maguire et al. 1996; Coulehan et al. 2001; Derksen et al. 2013; Kim et al. 2004). Empathetic doctors who are trusted by patients can provide comfort, hope and a sense of control to patients, however serious their disease (Montgomery 2006). Maxwell (2008) suggested that empathy could be seen as a core moral attribute. Hilfiker (2001) proposed that a fundamental goal of teaching ethics in medicine should be to foster empathy. Empathy broadly conceptualised becomes a way of seeing the world from the point of view of the patient, enabling students and doctors to perceive moral dimensions to clinical problems that they might otherwise ignore (Maxwell 2008).

There is some evidence that empathetic care results in less emotional distress, not only for patients, but also for doctors (Kearney et al. 2009; Jackson et al. 2008; Neumann et al. 2007; Hegazi and Wilson 2013; Larson and Yao 2005; Gleichgerrcht and Decety 2014). Jackson et al. (2008), in a qualitative study of oncologists' involvement in end-of-life care, showed that doctors who were connected to patients felt more fulfilled and had less burnout than colleagues who used distancing tactics.

Reiss acknowledged the benefits of empathy in clinical practice and questioned whether empathy must entail an emotional cost to healthcare professionals (Riess 2015). Batson suggests that empathy can be demonstrated as appropriate empathetic concern which need not necessarily include personal distress (Batson 2011). The context of the encounter may also contribute to emotional overload rather than fostering empathetic concern; for instance, if time is short or the workload excessive, emotional distress may follow (Gleichgerrcht and Decety 2013). Empathy in clinical practice has been described as 'emotional labour', which requires both effort and a conducive environment to achieve the best result (Riess 2015; Larson and Yao 2005).

Limits of Empathy

Although all students reported that empathy was central to their practice, some argued initially that the main priority of medicine was to improve the patient's condition.

Some authors have also expressed reservations about empathy. Macnaughton (2009) described empathy as 'dangerous' and warned of 'the way in which medicine can highjack complex ideas, confining them and defining them in its own terms and changing their meaning and impact'. She favoured a cognitive model of empathy arguing that in clinical practice, 'one person meets the other not as a fellow being but as a type of a person: as doctor or patient' (Macnaughton 2009). However, empathy can be seen as a mechanism for ensuring that a student or doctor regards the patient as a fellow human being, and not solely as an object of clinical interest. Macnaughton developed her argument by claiming that a full experience of mutuality or understanding of another person was not possible (Macnaughton 2009). The counterargument is that although a full understanding of another person may not be possible, this did not mean that people should be treated simply according to their role as patients in the clinical encounter (Halpern 2001). Halpern (2001) maintained that it was always possible, through adopting a broad open approach to empathy, to gain a better understanding of the patient's perspective.

Bloom (2016), in his book '*Against Empathy*', defined empathy in purely affective terms, then asserted that this narrowly defined empathy created a bias against patients. Instead, he proposed a form of 'rational compassion', which seemed similar to the broad form of empathy which included emotional elements. Critics of empathy tend to equate it with identification, but empathy, unlike identification, crucially retains a sense of a psychological boundary between the self and the other (Macnaughton 2009; Bondi 2003; Watson and Greenburg 2011).

Smajdor et al. (2011) also argued that emotional connection with the patient was unnecessary, suggesting that politeness was sufficient to meet the patient's needs. They justified this surprising claim by suggesting that objectivity protected the doctor and that distancing from the patient was therefore essential in medical practice (Smajdor et al. 2011). However, rather than enforcing a choice between objectivity and connection with a patient, the authors conceded that they might coexist by a switching between modes depending on the clinical context.

As Macnaughton suggested, there are limits to empathy, to understand others there is a need to consider a wider social and cultural context than can be supplied by empathy alone (Macnaughton 2009; Stueber 2006). Halpern proposed that doctors needed to approach this dilemma by being genuinely curious to learn more of the patient's experience (Halpern 2001). She argued that clinical curiosity can help to prevent doctors from being naively sympathetic or projecting their own concerns on the patient. This view of empathy as a form of engaged curiosity goes beyond surface emotions and seeks to understand the patient's experience, by adopting a phenomenological approach (Halpern 2014; Vagle 2016).

Evolution of Empathy

Theodor Lipps (1851–1914) adopted the term *Einfühlung* (feeling into) from aesthetics, to explain how people became aware of each other's mental states, with an emphasis on emotional (affective) aspects of empathy (Lipps 1903). *Einfühlung,* according to Lipps, was a process of imitation, or inner resonance, with the other person, an 'emotional contagion' (Lipps 1903). In 1909, Edward Tichener (1867–1927) used the Greek word *empatheia* to translate *Einfühlung* and was first to introduce the term 'empathy' (Tichner 1909).

From the outset, empathy was seen as essentially involving emotions. However, early in the twentieth century the concept of empathy became associated with the concept of understanding, '*verstehen*', in phenomenological philosophy. Phenomenologists such as Husserl (1859–1938), Stein (1891–1942) and Scheler (1874–1928) were concerned with the vexed question of intersubjectivity, the problem of other minds (Coplan and Goldie 2011). For Husserl, empathy was a unique mode of consciousness through which others' thoughts, emotions and desires were directly experienced, enabling others to be experienced as 'minded' (Husserl 1989; Stein 1989). Husserl described empathy as an understanding of the meaning of the other person's shared humanity (Hooker 2015).

Stein further developed the concept of empathy by postulating that it not only enabled us to understand others, but also to understand ourselves as others experience us, adding a relational dimension to empathy (Stein 1989). Stein described empathy as 'happening' to us, somewhat like falling in love, i.e. a process that could not be forced (Davis 1990). She outlined a process of empathy in three stages: seeing the world from the other person's point of view, a sudden 'crossing over' involving an emotional shift with deep understanding, and finally, regaining the self-other boundary (Stein 1989; Davis 1990).

From a clinical perspective, Carl Rogers (1899–1959), a founder of humanistic psychology, placed empathy at the heart of his patient-centred psychotherapy (Rogers 1961). Rogers claimed that empathy occurred when the therapist viewed patients with an 'unconditional positive regard' (Rogers 1959). He proposed that when we empathise, we enter the world of the other and become at home in it, thus stressing the relational nature of empathy (Rogers 1961). He pointed out the risk of over-identifying with the patient, maintaining that this could distort understanding and threaten the therapeutic process. He further argued that an empathetic encounter depended upon maintaining a 'self-other' distinction (Rogers 1961).

Martin Buber (1878–1965) was also influential in promoting the affective elements of empathy in his description of an 'I/Thou relationship', rather than the objective 'I/It' in a process he called 'dialogue' (Buber 2004). In the process of 'dialogue', one person becomes closely connected to the other in a moment of shared meaning (Buber 1961). Schutz (1899–1959) expanded the concept of empathy by focusing attention on the shared context where two subjects interact and affect each other in a face-to-face encounter, creating a 'we-relationship' (Schutz 1967).

These early, relational, affective views of empathy may be contrasted with the way in which empathy is now generally viewed in a medical context as a cognitive construct.

The Complexity of Empathy

Students talked about the complexity of empathy describing it in terms of a personal attribute (intrapersonal) and later, as a dynamic two-way relationship (interpersonal), which depended on the context of the patient–student consultation. They explored the practicalities of the process of empathising with a patient.

The students' stories revealed empathy to be a complex construct variously described as: feeling what another person feels, 'caring about others', imagining oneself in another's situation, having the capacity to grasp the content of other people's minds and as a virtue in response to suffering (Batson 2011; Coplan and Goldie 2011). The definition of empathy has consequences for patient care. If empathy is equated with detached concern, there is a risk of encouraging distancing behaviour in medical students (Hardy 2017).

Empathy as an Attribute (Intrapersonal)

Students in the first year shared a variety of notions of empathy as an attribute, a cognitive construct. They described empathy as trying to see the world from the patient's point of view.

> Empathy is trying to put yourself into someone else's shoes and experience essentially for yourself what it is like to be in that situation. But I think true empathy is trying to understand it from their side it's not about you but you are always the starting point. (Connie, Year 1)

It appeared from this account, that although empathy involved trying to see the world from the patient's perspective, the process starts with the empathiser, who is inevitably implicated in the encounter. Some students proposed that the cognitive dimension of empathy differentiated the construct from sympathy. They acknowledged limits to empathy, since it was not possible to know for certain what another person was thinking.

> interpret things from their point of view rather than feel sorry for them, which would be sympathy. (Gina, Year 3)

Students observed that some people seemed better at empathising than others. Kim linked this empathetic ability with their capacity for imagination, viewing empathy as a personal attribute.

> probably innate in that some people tend to have vivid imaginations and some people don't. (Kim, Year 4)

Empathy has largely been conceptualised in the medical education literature as an innate, personal attribute, subject to measurement (Baron-Cohen 2011; Hojat et al. 2009; Hojat 2016). In contrast to the early phenomenological approaches which emphasise the emotional, relational and contextual nature of empathy, medical practice has largely adopted a cognitive view of empathy. Hojat et al. (2009) defined empathy in purely cognitive terms. Hojat (2016), in advocating a cognitive view of empathy, claimed that by limiting empathy to its cognitive form enabled the construct to be studied and measured scientifically.

> Empathy is a predominantly cognitive (rather than emotional) attribute that involves an understanding (rather than feeling) of experiences, concerns and perspectives of the patient, combined with a capacity to communicate this understanding. An intention to help by preventing and alleviating pain and suffering is an additional feature of empathy in the context of patient care. (Hojat et al. 2009, p. 1183)

This view, which excludes emotions, perpetuates a form of medical professionalism which has been described as 'detached concern' (Fox and Lief 1963; Halpern 2001; Kelly 2017). A cognitive approach to empathy attempts to safeguard the objectivity and neutrality of scientific medical knowledge by depicting healthcare professionals' emotions as an undesirable bias, requiring cognitive control (Hojat 2016; Hooker 2015;

Pedersen 2009). In a recent review, Howick et al. suggest the term therapeutic empathy which includes an attempt to understand the patient's emotions without experiencing them (Howick et al. 2018a). However, one might imagine that it would be natural for doctors to adopt a form of empathy which included emotions, since much of medicine is concerned with the relief of suffering (Jeffrey 2016a).

In the preclinical years, many students viewed empathy as a static attribute which concurred with much of the medical education literature on empathy (Hojat et al. 2004; Neumann et al. 2012; Tavakol et al. 2012). An intrapersonal view of empathy underpins the theory behind most of the quantitative research directed at measuring empathy (Hojat et al. 2009). However, a static view of empathy does not clarify how empathy is experienced and disregards the impact of context on empathy (Marshall and Hooker 2016; Campos et al. 2011).

In the preclinical years, students also tended to describe empathy in terms of polarities, of affective and cognitive dimensions, a view often adopted in the literature (Baron-Cohen 2011; Hojat 2007). Hooker argued that framing the complexity of empathy in terms of polarities perpetuated the notion of scientific medicine as separate from and opposite to emotional care (Hooker 2015). While students understood the significance of cognitive aspects of empathy, they were uncertain about the extent to which they should share emotions with the patient. Eikeland et al. (2014) found that some students believed they should be like scientists, unbiased and capable of detached observation, with the result that some students in their study became cynical observers.

Maxwell (2008) suggested it was unhelpful to view cognitive and affective empathy as polarities. He argued that the emotional aspect of empathy inevitably contained a cognitive element, as it involved an intentional sharing of emotions and was not simply a reactive distress. Maxwell (2008) proposed that the contrast between affective and cognitive concepts of empathy should not create opposing views but rather reflect which dimension of clinical empathy predominated in any interaction. The cognitive-affective polarities of empathy need to be brought together to achieve appropriate empathetic care (Hooker 2015).

In contrast, the students in this study were convinced of the benefits of empathy in its broad dynamic form which included affective dimensions. They rejected the notion of a doctor as a cold detached observer of facts and were distressed when they saw such physicians in practice. Halpern, like the majority of students in this study, viewed empathy as essentially an affective mode of understanding, where the empathising student was moved by the patient's experience (Halpern 2003).

Empathy as a Relationship (Interpersonal)

The students described empathy as having affective, behavioural, moral and cognitive components. From a nursing perspective, Morse et al. (1992) divided the components of empathy into four dimensions:

- affective (the ability to subjectively experience and share in another's psychological state or feelings)
- cognitive (the ability to identify and understand another person's feelings and perspective from an objective stance)
- moral (an internal altruistic motivation)
- behavioural (communicating the response to convey understanding of another's perspective) (Morse et al. 1992).

Broad definitions of empathy propose that the doctor has to try to understand the patient's world, share their feelings and communicate this understanding to them (Irving and Dickson 2004; Derksen et al. 2013). Some authors have extended the broad view of empathy to include taking action to help the patient (Decety 2011). Mercer and Reynolds (2002) proposed such an expanded view of relational empathy, suggesting that empathy includes the ability to:

(a) understand the patient's situation, perspective and feelings (and their attached meanings)
(b) communicate that understanding and check its accuracy
(c) act on that understanding with the patient in a helpful (therapeutic) way (Mercer and Reynolds 2002).

However, Mercer and Reynolds (2002) did not clarify the extent of emotional sharing between the student and the patient. Does the student/doctor share the feelings of the patient, merely identify them, understand them or even ignore them? Halpern argued that a crucial a part of empathy was to recognise what it feels like to experience something rather than merely labelling an emotional state (Halpern 2003).

In the 1980s, second-wave feminist 'care ethics', added relational and moral dimensions to empathy, maintaining that moral thought and action required both reason and emotion in attempting to understand the situation from another person's point of view (Gilligan 1982; Noddings 1984; Slote 2007). From this perspective, to care for another involved 'feeling with' the other person, which resonated with the concept of *Einfühlung*, and a relational view of empathy (Lipps 1903; Stein 1989). Noddings proposed that when one empathises one becomes engrossed in the other person (Noddings 2013). Viewing empathy as a relational process is less common in the medical education literature (Evans 2012; Gerdes 2011; Halpern 2014). Taking a relational approach switches the focus of interest from the student's attributes to an exploration of the interaction between the student and patient. In this interaction, context becomes of particular significance. As Halpern (2014) suggested, there may be different empathies for specific clinical situations, depending upon the individual patient. She advocated that the student adopted a stance of 'engaged curiosity' in which understanding the patient's individual perspective was combined with emotionally engaged communication (Halpern 2014).

Affective (Emotional)

Although all students agreed that trying to understand the patients' view was their prime concern in empathising, there was less certainty when they came to discuss the emotional aspects of empathy. There were mixed views on whether it was appropriate to share feelings with the patient. Some students implied that empathy involved experiencing the patient's emotions. Others spoke of limiting emotional involvement to understanding the implications of the patient's feelings. Olive maintained that empathy involved a sharing of emotions and experiencing the feeling oneself, suggesting it was possible to know exactly how the other person was feeling. However, later she reflected on this view and suggested that some distance from the patient's emotion might be more appropriate. Other students argued that to understand a patient properly it was necessary to share feelings.

> I think it is just being able to put yourself in their shoes and know exactly how they are feeling and be able to take some of that upon yourself. And share whatever they are feeling. (Olive, Year 1)

> I would have to be able to understand properly what they are going through. I would have to try to imagine myself feeling some of their feelings. (Kim, Year 4)

Although many of the students suggested that sharing feelings with the patient was a part of empathy, they also were mindful that too much emotion might be overwhelming. Paula suggested that while it was appropriate to share the patient's feelings, it was not necessary to share the same intensity of emotion as that of the patient.

> I don't think you can be truly empathetic without [being] personally affected the way someone is feeling. Equally there is an element, you can't take on everything that the person is feeling. So you can be empathetic in being understanding toward them without necessarily feeling everything they feel. (Paula, Year 4)

However, in contrast, Marilyn advocated that doctors should remain detached from the emotions of the patient.

> Feeling what the patients feels no, no, no, no, no, no, no, no. So if we are going by that strict definition of empathy, don't do it! Don't do it. (Marilyn, Year 1)

The medical education literature reveals that students do not share a common understanding of empathy. In a Scandinavian study, it was reported that students viewed empathy as predominantly a cognitive construct which did not involve sharing feelings with a patient (Eikeland et al. 2014). In contrast, in another study, students suggested that empathy did involve connecting emotionally with the patient (Ratanawongsa et al. 2005). Students' views of empathy varied, some maintained that felt emotions would help them to be more effective doctors, while others defined empathy by contrasting it with sympathy.

Behavioural

The students attributed a behavioural quality to empathy, involving an action to help the patient. Diana linked empathy to altruism, as empathy engendered helpful action.

> doing something, something for somebody without necessarily without have any plans to get anything back from it. (Diana, Year 5)

Students also gave other examples of actions resulting from empathy; deciding how to present a treatment option to a patient or using empathy as a tool to aid patient compliance.

Moral

Students talked about empathy as a moral construct; as a motivating force to provide care; or as a virtue of a good doctor.

> if you say 'What qualities does a doctor need?' Empathy is always one of the words that comes up. (Fiona, Year 1)

In other studies, empathy has been described by students as a virtue, pointing to a need for humility and kindness in medical care (Eikeland et al. 2014; Ratanawongsa et al. 2005; Tavakol et al. 2012;

Nogucira-Martins et al. 2006). When a person acts morally, she has to consider the implications of her actions on the welfare of others (Cooper 2011). Thus ethics and empathy are inevitably interrelated (Hogan 1973).

Cognitive (Understanding)

Later in the course, cognitive understanding was described by the clinical students as an interpersonal activity. Both the student and the patient are engaged in a construction of meaning through an iterative process to gain understanding (Hooker 2015). Empathy cannot achieve an identical or complete understanding of the other person but, as Bondi (2014) argued, in reaching out and connecting with the other and accounting for differences in perspectives, empathy can be of great value. Students reflected this in their comments of the way in which empathy could spread through a team. They described empathy as a bridge between the doctor and the patient, equalising power between them, and so facilitating the patient to voice their deepest concerns. Shapiro (2008) argued that if working out how to bridge the inevitable distance between a doctor and a patient was at the heart of good medical practice, then empathy was the most important of the professional virtues.

From the students' accounts, empathy emerged as a multidimensional, dynamic concept which differed in various clinical situations, some students stressing understanding but for others, sharing feelings was paramount. They saw the various dimensions of empathy interacting but altering in emphasis according to the context of the relationship and the needs of the patient.

The students in the clinical years described empathy as a dynamic emotional resonance: a dialogue between themselves and the patient, a view supported by some authors (Halpern 2001; Main et al. 2017; Kupetz 2014). This view of empathy is also supported by Hollan (2008) and by Warmington (2012) who claimed that there was a need for ongoing dialogue for true empathy. Warmington (2012) described these processes as 'attentiveness' and respectful dialogue. A relational view of empathy acknowledged that the emotions and thoughts of one person influenced the other in a two-way process and was affected by the context of their encounter (Campos et al. 2011; Hooker 2015).

The Process of Empathising

The commonest perspective amongst the students in the clinical group was of empathy as a relational process, rather than as a personal attribute. Empathy between two people was seen as being influenced by the context of the relationship.

> empathy takes two people and even if one person is the same, changing the other person is going to change the way that they are empathizing. (Connie, Year 2)

Students explored this dynamic process by describing a series of steps which might be involved, beginning a willingness to empathise with the patient.

Approachability

All students expressed a willingness to empathise. They described this as being interested to learn more about the patient in a collaboration.

> ask what her concerns are?, what does she want to know?, what her understanding was at that point of time? Can we can we work together on this? (Neville, Year 4)

They maintained that first impressions were the basis for establishing empathy, implying that patients made a rapid judgement as to how approachable they found the student. Students described how a warm empathetic greeting could set the tone for the whole consultation with the patient and establish rapport.

Listening

Students suggested that empathy could be established merely by being present and prepared to spend time with the patient. Amy explained how she abandoned her medical agenda to sit listen to the patient.

> I just put my pen and paper aside, and stop writing every single thing, frantically trying to scribble all the history. I just thought OK, I'm going to listen to her and then she opened up, and she cried. (Amy, Year 4)

Students described empathetic listening as a key part of forming a connection with patients. Gina suggested that it also involved demonstrating to the patient that you have heard their concerns.

> being empathic and listening other patient they need to know that you have been doing that, to really feel like they have gotten something out of the consultation. (Gina, Year 5)

Since students had emphasised the necessity for listening to the patient they described feeling distressed when pressure of time did not permit this. In this situation they found that they had to balance their empathy with a competing demand to be efficient; they described a tension between empathy and efficiency. This tension was one of the major themes discussed by the students during the research.

> I would love to sit and listen, listen to that person. It is always finding that balance of efficiency, professionalism, making sure the patient is safe and also being a good human being. (Neville, Year 6)

Emotions

In the next step of empathising, the students discussed whether it was appropriate to share their feelings with the patient. Most students said that feelings were an integral part of empathy and should involve not just identifying and understanding the patient's emotion but also sharing it to a degree. Some suggested that it was appropriate sometimes to show their feelings.

> I think it is important that they [patients] know that it has affected you. (Edward, Year 1)

Connie questioned whether it was even possible to understand an emotion without feeling it, implying that empathy could be emotionally exhausting and may require effort. She reflected how the patient viewed an empathetic doctor, proposing that sharing feelings was a way of demonstrating that she cared. She reflected on empathy as a response which acknowledged the other person and opened up opportunities to help the patient.

> it is about a response that lets them know you understand not just academically but you can personally connect with their situation. Which then opens up a number of opportunities for[...]for help. (Connie, Year 2)

On the other hand, Fiona exemplified the ambiguity many students felt about sharing feelings, initially arguing that it was not necessary to experience the patient's emotions, but a year later, describing emotions as being innate and shared.

> to be empathetic I don't think you have to take on the feelings as such. You have to understand them in order than to take right actions appropriately. (Fiona, Year 2)

Neville claimed that he had to experience the patient's emotions to be a good doctor, using the metaphor of a roller coaster. He also maintained that the student need not experience the same intensity of the emotion as the patient.

> Unless you do that, unless you feel that roller coaster I don't think you are a good doctor. (Neville, Year 5)

Kim described a more sophisticated process of switching between different forms of empathy, cognitive and affective, adapting the form of empathy to the needs of the individual patient.

> I think to be able to empathise properly with that person there has to be an emotional component [...] I suppose you can switch between the two [...] If you go and see a patient you can apply a different method depending what is necessary for that patient. (Kim, Year 4)

Some students like Marilyn expressed concerns about sharing emotions. Ida suggested that her role was to support the patient and was concerned that by sharing feelings she might burden the patient. Diana reflected that trying to control emotions completely would have a psychological cost to her.

> if I feel that patient would benefit from me showing that I really care then I might express that but I would be rather careful with it. (Marilyn, Year 2)

> because they already have so much burden themselves I don't want them to feel like have to take care of me because it should be the other way around. (Ida, Year 6)

> It is going to build up eventually isn't it?[...] There is no point being like an emotionless almost a robot. (Diana, Year 5)

Vulnerability

Many of the students said that to be empathetic involved exposing some of their vulnerability. They suggested that they should act in a natural, friendly manner on the same level as their patients. They implied that doctors needed some common humanity and to be prepared to share their vulnerability, and claimed that patients appreciated doctors who were prepared to do this

> anytime you show emotional connection with another person you have in some way invested the way you feel in the way that they feel. That does to some extent put you, well make you vulnerable. (Connie, Year 2)

Other students admitted that their own lack of life experience and knowledge made them feel unsure. However, Fiona pointed out that vulnerability could sometimes be an advantage, by placing the student on the same level as a patient, it could facilitate empathy.

> or you can turn it on head and say actually if you don't have as much knowledge you are exactly same level as the patient. (Fiona, Year 2)

Others suggested that some patients might be disturbed by a doctor showing vulnerability, but Olive said that she preferred a doctor to be open, suggesting that this might lead to more understanding.

> If a patient is wanting their doctor to be completely bullet proof and all that kind of stuff it won't help the patient for them to know actually that their doctors vulnerable too. But I think personally I would appreciate [the doctor] being open about that. (Olive, Year 1)

The students suggested that one way of sharing vulnerability was self-disclosure about their own experiences of illness. Olive warned that although this could be helpful, she could see dangers in making assumptions. In the clinical years, students became even more cautious about using self-disclosure, perhaps wishing to avoid burdening the patient.

> I think it can be really helpful for some patients. I don't think it needs to be I had this exact same disease either. (Olive, Year 1)

> I have stopped doing, I used to share quite a lot of my own stories from own view point in order to kind of get a connection with people. (Jenny, Year 4)

Kim recognised that there was a balance to be achieved, that some self-disclosure might help to establish empathy but there was a difference between the patient–doctor relationship and that of friendship. Friends often shared their personal information, but patients knew little about their doctors' personal lives.

> With the doctor patient relationship it is quite difficult in a way because as doctor you got to know a lot about that patient but they don't necessarily know very much about you at all. (Kim, Year 4)

Non-judgemental

Students maintained that they should strive to be non-judgemental and suggested that patients may confide more in them as students rather than doctors. Students found some patients were easier to empathise with than others, but felt obliged to try to empathise with every patient, as it affected the quality of care.

> if patients are nicer patients, if they are friendly to you and everyone around, it is easier to want to empathise with them, see their perspective and really address their needs. Obviously you still have to try even if you don't like a patient it can't influence your care. (Gina, Year 4)

Confronted with patients whose illness was due to an unhealthy lifestyle, Fiona distinguished between an initial 'gut reaction' to such patients, and a more reflective stance, which considered the possible reasons for their unhealthy behaviour. Marilyn thought she would become more judgemental as the course progressed and was surprised that she had not.

> your first gut reaction is yes this is because of life choices but then your second level of thinking is actually how free they were to make those choices? (Fiona, Year 1)

> I thought I would slowly develop a distaste for certain people, for groups of people, who drink and smoke and are obese and don't even try and then come in for this and that. (Marilyn, Year 2)

The students identified patients with a number of clinical conditions which challenged their empathy and their need to be non-judgemental. These patients, who both challenged and developed their empathy, are described in Chapter 7.

Continuity of Care

Olive argued for the need for continuity in her relationship with a patient. Gina reflected on the difficulty of gaining an idea of the patient's experience from the brief 'snapshot' she saw of them in the clinic. Paula expressed her sense of job satisfaction in having good relationships with patients.

> I think the continuous relationship is important and I think you can become more empathetic with people you know better. (Olive, Year 1)

> it is very fulfilling interacting with people that is what is enjoyable about the job. (Paula, Year 5)

It seems that deeper levels of empathy require not only individual attention and time but also some continuity in the relationship (Cooper 2011).

Understanding

Students identified two stances for taking a perspective on the patient's world, either a self- or an other-orientated perspective. Students felt that empathy should involve taking the patient's perspective (other-orientated). Since, as Fiona argued, it would not necessarily help a patient for her to imagine how she would feel in their situation.

> there is no point in how you would, as in I would feel in that position because that is not going to help me treat that person better. (Fiona, Year 1)

Gina reflected that although she tried to take an other-orientated perspective, she tended initially to take a self-orientated view. Other students described a sense of being overwhelmed in empathising when they thought, 'what this would be like for me?' It appeared that taking such a self-orientated perspective could cause personal distress.

> you are trying to put it from their perspective but actually thinking how you would feel in that situation. (Gina, Year 4)

> Sometimes I just find yourself imagining, What if I had that? (Paula, Year 4)

> I think it is not appropriate to imagine yourself in their place because that will mess you right up. It is not appropriate to look at a dying cancer patient and think 'Oh my God, what if that was me?' (Marilyn, Year 1)

Students were concerned not to project their own view on to the patient but tried to imagine things from the patient's perspective. Olive described this imaginative process as 'getting it'.

> I think it is very important to find out what's the priority, what the patient actually wants rather than what you want. (Amy, Year 4)

> I don't have to force myself to do all of this because I am on a ward and I 'get it'[…] So even though I don't have Mr Smith in front of me who has COPD, I can see how breathless he is. I can imagine. (Olive, Year 3)

Kim reflected on the role of her personal experience of illness in her perspective-taking in empathy, claiming that empathy was possible without having had the same experience as the patient. Paula suggested that empathising involved a pause, a step back, to try to appreciate the wider picture.

> I think empathy is where, without necessarily being through the situation yourself, you are able to understand what other people are going through and have some insight into how they are feeling and what they are thinking. (Kim, Year 4)

> sometimes to make a good clinical judgment maybe it is better to just look at the whole picture and step back and how you feel about it in order to be analytical and find the right solution. (Paula, Year 5)

These perspectives were further developed by Coplan and Goldie (2011), who viewed empathy as a unique kind of understanding through which we experienced what it was like to be another person, including their emotions, while maintaining a clear self-other differentiation. Empathy involved using one's imagination, which could be 'self'- or 'other'-orientated (Coplan and Goldie 2011).

In taking a self-orientated perspective, I imagine what it is like for me to be in your situation, a form of identification (Bondi 2014). Doctors who take a self-orientated perspective are at risk not only of personal distress, but compassion fatigue and eventually burnout (Kearney et al. 2009). In contrast, taking an other-orientated perspective, as in empathy, involves imagining undergoing the patient's experience (Halpern 2001).

This more sophisticated approach requires mental flexibility and an ability to regulate one's emotions. Bondi (2003) emphasised the importance of maintaining a self-other boundary, in a process of switching between observation and participation. Taking an other-orientated perspective prevents the doctor from losing sight of the patient as another person, despite having a deep engagement with them (Rogers 1961; Coplan and Goldie 2011).

The process of empathy has been described as a performance, rather similar to surface acting, exhibiting empathetic postures without engaging in feelings (Larson and Yao 2005). However, in my study most students described empathy as a means of gaining a special depth of understanding of patients, not from a detached external position, but from a more engaged stance of participant-observer, entering into the patient's lifeworld (Hooker 2015). This was reflected both by their interest in the process of empathising and by their wishes to connect with patients, a finding reflected in another phenomenological study (Tavakol et al. 2012). Svenaeus (2015) also maintained that empathy depended upon on the willingness of an individual to take an interest in the other person.

It seemed from the students' accounts that empathy required face-to-face contact with another person and that first impressions were central to this, ideas which accord with Lipps' original concept of *Einfühlung* (Lipps 1903). Suchman et al. (1997) described this initial contact with a patient as an 'empathic opportunity', while Barrett-Lennard (1981) termed the initial concern 'empathic resonation'. Some students in the clinical years pointed out that this resonation might occur by merely being present with the patient, reflecting the concept of 'attentiveness' in empathy described by Warmington (2012). Attentiveness involved the student's openness both to the patient's feelings and to their own emotions (Warmington 2012). Norfolk et al. (2007) described a relational model of empathy for developing rapport with patients in which they depicted empathy as a skill. Their model also highlighted the students' innate interest in the patient and their motivation to care for them which can be described as empathetic concern (Norfolk et al. 2007).

Batson (2011) captured the complexity of empathy by identifying eight related but distinct phenomena which are described as 'empathies' in the literature. He described the following eight 'empathies' before discussing the actual process of empathising with another person:

1. Knowing another person's internal state, including thoughts and feelings: sometimes described as cognitive empathy (Wispé 1986)
2. Adopting the posture of an observed other: motor mimicry (Lipps 1903)
3. Coming to feel as another person feels: affective empathy, emotional contagion or sympathy (Hoffman 2000)
4. Projecting oneself into another's situation: an aesthetic projection described as *Einfühlung* (Lipps 1903)
5. Imaging how another is thinking or feeling: other-orientated perspective-taking (Batson et al. 1991)
6. Imagining how one would think and feel in the other's place: self-orientated perspective-taking (Batson et al. 1997)
7. Feeling distress at witnessing another's suffering, personal distress (Batson and Shaw 1991)
8. Feeling for another person who is suffering, empathic concern (Batson 2011).

Batson's eight phenomena, each a form of empathy, provide a helpful basis for investigating the process of empathising (Batson 2011). The first six concepts are related to the question of how we know another person's thoughts. The last two concepts (concepts 7 and 8) are reactions to this knowledge, reflecting a caring response to suffering. It is not only other-orientated feelings (concept 8) which are a source of a caring response. A sensitive response may result from feeling as the other (concept 3), combined with an other-orientated perspective (concept 5) (Batson 2011).

Batson's model is helpful in distinguishing appropriate empathetic concern (concept 8) from harmful personal distress (concept 7) (Batson 2011). Empathetic concern is needed in clinical care and does not lead to burnout, whereas personal distress may result in distancing from the patient (Batson and Shaw 1991). Batson (2011) claimed that taking a self-orientated perspective risked causing personal distress. In contrast, taking an other-orientated perspective was necessary for appropriate empathetic concern.

A new insight was also gained from students who suggested that empathy involved action to help the suffering patient (Håkansson and Montgomery 2003). Motivation to act is thought by some authors to be a feature of compassion which differentiated it from empathy (Chochinov 2007). However in my study, students saw empathy as both a motivating force and a practical action, thus moving beyond Batson's empathy-altruism binary towards a view of empathy as a response to suffering (Batson 2011). Expanding the concept of empathy to include action to relieve suffering maintains the focus on the patient rather than the student and takes account of the social context of the patient's illness (Garden 2009). Garden (2009) suggested that recognising a patient's suffering was a starting point for empathy with action, in which the student explored the patient's experience of illness and their social situation, before acting with them to alleviate suffering. Warmington (2012) also claimed that an empathetic response involved both engagement and a commitment to help the patient.

In the literature, empathy is often conflated with compassion, sympathy and other prosocial behaviours, which further contributed to the difficulty in defining the construct.

Sympathy, Compassion and Other Prosocial Behaviours

To establish the focus on empathy in my book, I briefly review some of the main constructs which overlap with empathy in the literature (Jeffrey 2016c).

Sympathy has been defined as experiencing another's emotions, as opposed to imagining those emotions and as a concern for the welfare of others (Stepien and Baernstein 2006; Decety et al. 2010). Some authors argue that sympathy is a wholly distinct concept from empathy (Mercer and Reynolds 2002; Hojat 2016). However, I agree with those who argue that sympathy overlaps with the emotional component of empathy (Halpern 2001). Although sympathy is related to affective elements of empathy, it differs in that does not take an 'other-orientated' perspective. Sympathy takes a 'self-orientated' perspective, with identification with the other, which puts the listener at risk of personal distress (Batson 2011).

Compassion shares many features of empathy and has been described as 'a feeling of deep sympathy and sorrow for another who is stricken by suffering or misfortune, accompanied by a strong desire to alleviate the pain or remove its cause' (Von Dietze and Orb 2000). Since empathy is often confused with compassion in the medical literature, Maxwell (2008), suggested using the term 'compassionate empathy' to capture the imaginative connotations of empathy and a feeling of distress in solidarity with the patient. Compassion, in its drive to alleviate suffering, also shares elements of altruism, although in many definitions of compassion a cognitive dimension is missing (Von Dietze and Orb 2000). Confusing the definitions of empathy and compassion is unhelpful to medical research and practice and highlights the need for a common nomenclature (Howick and Rees 2017; Riess 2015).

Altruism is a motivation that is other-directed and manifested as an action (Burks and Kobus 2012). Altruistic behaviours are often described as 'going the extra mile' (Stocks et al. 2009). Batson proposes an altruism-empathy hypothesis suggesting that empathy often evokes altruistic behaviour (Batson et al. 1991).

Emotional intelligence is a concept which comprises: self-awareness, managing emotions appropriately, motivating oneself, recognising emotions in others (a form of empathy) and handling relationships. Emotional intelligence therefore includes empathy but also embodies other psychological and behavioural concepts (Goleman 1996).

Kindness may also involve empathy, but in modern life there has been a tendency to disparage kindness as being hopelessly idealistic and ineffectual (Philips and Taylor 2009). However, others have argued that kindness in a medical setting is no soft option, but inspires doctors to build relationships with patients and to treat them well (Ballatt and Campling 2011; Jeffrey 2016b).

Generosity, a willingness to give of oneself, is also related to empathy and may be manifest in several ways in clinical practice: openness to others, providing comfort and a commitment to not abandoning the patient (Frank 2004).

Resilience has been described as a dynamic capability which may include empathy and which allows people to thrive on challenges (Howe et al. 2012). Resilience includes capabilities such as self-control, a willingness to engage support and persistence. It has been described as a key attribute in preventing burnout (Howe et al. 2012).

A broad view of the term 'empathy' is better suited than 'compassion' for medical education, research and practice. It has been researched in greater depth in the medical education literature and because empathy retains a cognitive component which compassion may lack (Jeffrey 2016c).

Levels of Empathy

Students suggested that empathy could also be expressed at different levels. After their first exams, they described a superficial level of empathy as 'fake' empathy. In this situation, the student displayed behaviours such as body language or tone of voice which suggested they were being empathetic but in fact they were not attempting to see the world from the patient's point of view. Such 'fake' empathy might, for example, be displayed in exams with simulated patients such as the objective structured clinical examination (OSCE).

> we know that people are going to be looking for it when we are examined and that we need to clearly demonstrate it. (Connie, Year 2)

Although most students agreed that empathy could be faked, they emphasised that it was only valued when it was authentic. They argued that patients would soon detect 'fake' empathy, suggesting that a genuine approach would lead to a deeper understanding of the patient's needs, and to the delivery of appropriate care.

> if it is actually genuine then it will give you just a whole other level of understanding and hopefully that will give you a whole other level of treatment. (Olive, Year 2)

However, one student took a different view, claiming that as long as the patient felt that she was empathised with, then the authenticity of the empathy did not matter. She seemed to be suggesting that as long as the patient feels cared for it is less relevant what the doctor feels, so disregarding feelings of job satisfaction. For Marilyn, it was the patient's condition which was paramount.

> If you can behave empathetically and your patient feels happy, if your patient feels supported, if your patient feels you care. What you get is of no consequence. (Marilyn, Year 2)

In the clinical years, students talked of another level of empathy, of detached concern, in which the cognitive elements of empathy predominated and affective elements were absent. Kim described seeing consultants who appeared to be detached from the patient.

> I see other extremes of practice where they don't introduce their name, themselves and they just go in. (Kim, Year 4)

Students also described a 'deeper' level of empathy which involved a greater understanding and a sharing of emotions.

> I think that empathy [involves] just [that] extra level of understanding, more emotions. (Fiona, Year 2)

Some students reflected that these levels of empathy might be adapted to meet differing clinical contexts and the individual patient's needs and they noticed that this adaptation does not always occur.

> Not every patient wants the same thing, so we as doctors need to be adaptable and I think because we are not always aware of the patient experience, we have our way of doing things and we do that for all patients. (Gina, Year 6)

As they moved through the course, the students also described differing levels of empathy which varied according to the context. Bayne et al. (2013)

developed a relational model of empathy in which they differentiated two levels of empathy, initial empathy, which was exemplified by customer service, and genuine empathy, that was applicable to holistic care. Halpern considered levels of empathy by describing differing empathies for differing clinical contexts (Halpern 2014).

At one end of a spectrum of empathy, students described 'fake' empathy in OSCE exams where they showed empathetic behaviours without trying to understand the patient's view. Jamison (2014) pointed out the difference between being assessed for empathy and the nuanced nature of true empathy in practice. Indeed, students described how their genuine empathy diminished when they were being assessed. Other students have described how empathy risks being reduced to simply another communication skill (Light et al. 2018). Fake empathy has been compared to surface acting in which empathetic expressions are adopted without any change in the student's emotions or understanding of the patient (Larson and Yao 2005). Students described the next level of empathy as 'detached concern' which did not attempt to make an emotional connection with the patient (Halpern 2001). Agosta took a stronger position by dismissing detached concern as being a professionally motivated lack of empathy (Agosta 2014).

In contrast, authentic empathy was at the other end of the spectrum. Only one student argued that as long as the patient felt cared for, the feelings of the student or doctor were irrelevant. The others maintained that patients would detect empathy which was not genuine. Authenticity seems more akin to deep acting where the actor feels the emotions rather than merely altering their emotional expressions (Larson and Yao 2005). Larson claimed that the scope of empathy goes far beyond the communication skills of surface acting (Larson and Yao 2005). True empathy involved connecting with the patient both cognitively and emotionally, acting to help the patient with a feeling of responsibility for their duty of care (Macintyre 1985). True empathy was not only a sharing of feelings and understanding, but it was also a way of responding to the patient (Svenaeus 2015). Empathy conceptualised at this level involved recognition of the patient as a fellow human being and developing a sense of fraternity. Agosta (2014) described this deep form of empathy as enabling one person to humanise the other by recognising and acknowledging the possibilities for transformation and healing in the other. This feeling of a shared humanity can create a sense of security in situations of great uncertainty, for instance, in end-of-life care (Svenaeus 2014).

Cooper proposed three levels of empathy; fundamental, profound and functional (Cooper 2011). Fundamental empathy consists of the interest in the other person and the communication skills facilitating empathy. Profound empathy corresponds with the broad or deep form described by the students. It embraces emotions, self-awareness, relationships and moral aspects of empathy. Functional empathy is involved in working with groups of people rather than individuals (Cooper 2011). Cooper proposes that when people are treated as numbers as opposed to unique human beings emotional aspects of empathy are lost (Cooper 2011).

Context of Empathy

In contrast to descriptions of empathy in the literature, the students emphasised the influence of context on the empathetic process (Marshall and Hooker 2016). In discussing the process of empathy in the context of clinical practice, the debate moves beyond arguments over how this complex concept should be defined into deeper thinking about the nature of the patient–student relationship (Marshall and Hooker 2016; Derksen et al. 2013; Irving and Dickson 2004; Coplan and Goldie 2011).

Empathy is often described in the literature as something which occurs between a doctor and a patient but not as something which is influenced by time, location or other aspects of context (Marshall and Hooker 2016). In contrast, the students have emphasised the central importance of context in descriptions of empathising with patients. Therefore, this phenomenological study is less concerned with what characteristics the students 'have', but rather focuses on what happens in the student–patient relationship: the process of empathising (Marshall and Hooker 2016).

The students' relational perspective of empathy developed with their contact with patients and reflected Stein's early phenomenological work on relational empathy (Stein 1989). Students' views moved beyond the polarities of affective and cognitive domains to integrate behavioural and moral facets of empathy which interacted in differing ways depending on the patient's needs and the context of the situation (Sulzer et al. 2016). The students' stories suggested that empathy was something they did, rather than something they had (Marshall and Hooker 2016; Zaki and Williams 2013).

A relational view of empathy implied that the student's success in empathising with a patient partially depended on the openness of patient and on the context of their meeting (Halpern 2001; Main et al. 2017). Feedback from the patient can help a student to develop a greater understanding of the patient's lifeworld, and this was reflected in the students' views on the value of continuity to empathy (Main et al. 2017). Some students claimed that their lack of life experience sometimes limited their ability to empathise. However, this implied that the patient's experiences were understood from the student's perspective rather than that of the patient (Hardy 2017). Gallagher suggested that students need narrative competency which allowed them to interact with the patient in a joint process of making sense of the world (Gallagher 2012; Hardy 2017).

Students talked about a number of contexts in which their empathy was constrained: environment, time, lack of continuity, stress and competition. These issues are discussed fully in Chapters 6 and 7.

Key Points

Three major themes relating to the process of empathising emerged from the students' conversations;

- their perceived risks of emotional connection with patients,
- detachment as a coping mechanism,
- how to regulate emotions.

References

Agosta, L. (2014). A rumor of empathy: Reconstructing Heidegger's contribution to empathy and empathic clinical practice. *Medicine, Health Care and Philosophy, 17,* 281–292.

Balint, M. (1957). *The Doctor His Patient and the Illness.* London: Tavistock Publications.

Ballatt, J., & Campling, P. (2011). *Intelligent Kindness.* London: RCPsych Publications.

Baron-Cohen, S. (2011). *Zero Degrees of Empathy.* London: Allen Lane.

Barrett-Lennard, G. T. (1981). The empathy cycle: Refinement of a nuclear concept. *Journal of Counseling Psychology, 28,* 91–100.

Batson, C. (2011). These things called empathy: Eight related but distinct phenomena. In J. Decety & W. Ickes (Eds.), *The Social Neuroscience of Empathy.* Cambridge: MIT Press.

Batson, C. D., & Shaw, L. L. (1991). Evidence for altruism: Toward a pluralism of prosocial motives. *Psychological Inquiry, 2,* 107–122.

Batson, C. D., Early, S., & Salvarani, G. (1997). Perspective taking: Imagining how another feels versus imaging how you would feel. *Personality and Social Psychology Bulletin, 23,* 751–758.

Batson, C. D., Batson, J. G., Slingsby, J., Harrell, K. L., Peekna, H. M., & Todd, R. M. (1991). Empathic joy and the empathy-altruism hypothesis. *Journal of Personality and Social Psychology, 61,* 413–426.

Bayne, H., Neukrug, E., Hays, D., & Britton, B. (2013). A comprehensive model for optimizing empathy in person-centered care. *Patient Education and Counseling, 93,* 209–215.

Bloom, P. (2016). *Against Empathy: The Case for Rational Compassion.* London: The Bodley Head.

Bondi, L. (2003). Empathy and identification: Conceptual resources for feminist fieldwork. *ACME: An International E-Journal for Critical Geographies, 2,* 64–76.

Bondi, L. (2014). Understanding feelings: Engaging with unconscious communication and embodied knowledge. *Emotion, Space and Society, 10,* 44–54.

Broyard, A. (1992). *Intoxicated by My Illness: And Other Writings on Life and Death.* New York: Fawcett Columbine.

Buber, M. (1961). *Between Man and Man.* London: Collins.

Buber, M. (2004). *I and Thou.* London: Continuum.

Burks, D. J., & Kobus, A. M. (2012). The legacy of altruism in health care: The promotion of empathy, prosociality and humanism. *Medical Education, 46,* 317–325.

Campos, J. J., Walle, E. A., Dahl, A., & Main, A. (2011). Reconceptualizing emotion regulation. *Emotion Review, 3,* 26–35.

Chochinov, H. (2007). Dignity and the essence of medicine: The A, B, C, and D of dignity conserving care. *British Medical Journal, 335,* 184–187.

Cooper, B. (2011). *Empathy in Education: Engagement, Values and Achievement.* London: Bloomsbury Publishing.

Coplan, A., & Goldie, P. (Eds.). (2011). *Empathy: Philosophical and Psychological Perspectives.* Oxford: Oxford University Press.

Coulehan, J. L., Platt, F. W., Egener, B., Frankel, R., Lin, C.-T., Lown, B., et al. (2001). "Let me see if I have this right…": Words that help build empathy. *Annals of Internal Medicine, 135,* 221–227.

Coulter, A. (2002). Patients' views of the good doctor. *British Medical Journal, 325,* 668–669.

Davis, C. M. (1990). What is empathy, and can empathy be taught? *Physical Therapy, 70,* 707–711.

Decety, J. (2011). *Empathy: From Bench to Bedside.* Cambridge: MIT Press.

Decety, J., Yang, C.-Y., & Cheng, Y. (2010). Physicians down-regulate their pain empathy response: An event-related brain potential study. *Neuroimage, 50,* 1676–1682.

del Canale, S., Louis, D., Maio, V., Wang, X., Rossi, G., Hojat, M., et al. (2012). The relationship between physician empathy and disease complications: An empirical study of primary care physicians and their diabetic patients in Parma, Italy. *Academic Medicine, 87,* 1243–1249.

Derksen, F., Bensing, J., & Lagro-Janssen, A. (2013). Effectiveness of empathy in general practice: A systematic review. *British Journal General Practice, 63,* 76–84.

di Blasi, Z., Harkness, E., Ernst, E., Georgiou, A., & Kleijnen, J. (2001). Influence of context effects on health outcomes: A systematic review. *The Lancet, 357,* 757–762.

Eikeland, H. L., Ornes, K., Finset, A., & Pedersen, R. (2014). The physician's role and empathy—A qualitative study of third year medical students. *BMC Medical Education, 14,* 165–173.

Evans, M. (2012). Feeling my way: Emotions and empathy in geographic research with fathers in Valparaíso, Chile. *Area, 44,* 503–509.

Fox, R., & Lief, H. (1963). Training for "detached concern". In H. Lief (Ed.), *The Psychological Basis of Medical Practice.* New York: Harper Row.
Frank, A. (2004). *The Renewal of Generosity.* Chicago: University of Chicago Press.
Gallagher, S. (2012). Empathy, simulation, and narrative. *Science in Context, 25,* 355–381.
Garden, R. (2009). Expanding clinical empathy: An activist perspective. *Journal of General Internal Medicine, 24,* 122–125.
General Medical Council. (2009). *Tomorrow's Doctors: Outcomes and Standards for Undergraduate Medical Education.* London: General Medical Council.
General Medical Council. (2013). *Good Medical Practice.* London: General Medical Council.
General Medical Council. (2015). *Outcomes for Graduates (Tomorrow's Doctors).* London: General Medical Council.
Gerdes, K. (2011). Empathy, sympathy, and pity: 21st-century definitions and implications for practice and research. *Journal of Social Service Research, 37,* 230–241.
Gilligan, C. (1982). *In a Different Voice: Psychological Theory and Womens' Development.* Cambridge: Harvard University Press.
Gleichgerrcht, E., & Decety, J. (2013). Empathy in clinical practice: How individual dispositions, gender, and experience moderate empathic concern, burnout, and emotional distress in physicians. *PLoS ONE* [Online], *8.* Available http://journals.plos.org/plosone/article/file?id=10.1371/journal.pone.0061526&type=printable. Accessed January 29, 2018.
Gleichgerrcht, E., & Decety, J. (2014). The relationship between different facets of empathy, pain perception and compassion fatigue among physicians. *Frontiers in Behavioral Neuroscience, 8,* 1–9.
Goleman, D. (1996). *Emotional Intelligence: Why Can It Matter More Than IQ?* London: Bloomsbury Publishing.
Håkansson, J., & Montgomery, H. (2003). Empathy as an interpersonal phenomenon. *Journal of Social and Personal Relationships, 20,* 267–284.
Halpern, J. (2001). *From Detached Concern to Empathy: Humanizing Medical Practice.* Oxford: Oxford University Press.
Halpern, J. (2003). What is clinical empathy? *Journal of General Internal Medicine, 18,* 670–674.
Halpern, J. (2012). Gathering the patient's story and clinical empathy. *The Permanente Journal, 16,* 1.
Halpern, J. (2014). From idealized clinical empathy to empathic communication in medical care. *Medicine, Health Care and Philosophy, 17,* 301–311.

Hardy, C. (2017). Empathizing with patients: The role of interaction and narratives in providing better patient care. *Medicine, Healthcare and Philosophy.*, *20,* 237–248.

Hegazi, I., & Wilson, I. (2013). Maintaining empathy in medical school: It is possible. *Medical Teacher, 35,* 1002–1008.

Hilfiker, D. (2001). From the victim's point of view. *Journal of Medical Humanities, 22,* 255–263.

Hoffman, M. (2000). *Empathy and Moral Development: Implications for Caring and Justice.* Cambridge: Cambridge University Press.

Hogan, R. (1973). Moral conduct and moral character: A psychological perspective. *Psychological Bulletin, 79,* 217.

Hojat, M. (2007). *Empathy in Patient Care: Antecedents, Development, Measurement, and Outcomes.* New York: Springer.

Hojat, M. (2016). *Empathy in Health Profession Education and Primary Care.* New York: Springer.

Hojat, M., Louis, D. Z., Markham, F. W., Wender, R., Rabinowitz, C., & Gonnella, J. (2011). Physicians' empathy and clinical outcomes for diabetic patients. *Academic Medicine, 86,* 359–364.

Hojat, M., Mangione, S., Nasca, T. J., Rattner, S., Erdmann, J. B., Gonnella, J. S., et al. (2004). An empirical study of decline in empathy in medical school. *Medical Education, 38,* 934–941.

Hojat, M., Vergare, M. J., Maxwell, K., Brainard, G., Herrine, S. K., Isenberg, G. A., et al. (2009). The devil is in the third year: A longitudinal study of erosion of empathy in medical school. *Academic Medicine, 84,* 1182–1191.

Hollan, D. (2008). Being there: On the imaginative aspects of understanding others and being understood. *Ethos, 36,* 475–489.

Hooker, C. (2015). Understanding empathy: Why phenomenology and hermeneutics can help medical education and practice. *Medicine, Health Care and Philosophy, 18,* 541–552.

Howe, A., Smajdor, A., & Stöckl, A. (2012). Towards an understanding of resilience and its relevance to medical training. *Medical Education, 46,* 349–356.

Howick, J., & Rees, S. (2017). Overthrowing barriers to empathy in healthcare: Empathy in the age of the internet. *Journal of the Royal Society of Medicine, 110,* 1–6.

Howick, J., Bizzari, V., & Dambha-Miller, H. (2018a). Therapeutic empathy: What it is and what it isn't. *Journal of the Royal Society of Medicine, 111,* 233–236.

Howick, J., Moscrop, A., Mebius, A., Fanshawe, T. R., Lewith, G., & Bishop, F. L., et al. (2018b). Effects of empathic and positive communication in healthcare consultations: A systematic review and meta-analysis. *Journal of the Royal Society of Medicine*. https://doi.org/10.1177/0141076818769477.

Husserl, E. (1989). *Ideas Pertaining to a Pure Phenomenology and to a Phenomenological Philosophy. Second Book: Studies in the Phenomenology of Constitution*. Dordrecht: Kluwer Academic Publishers.

Irving, P., & Dickson, D. (2004). Empathy: Towards a conceptual framework for health professionals. *International Journal of Health Care Quality Assurance, 17,* 212–220.

Jackson, V., Mack, J., Matsuyama, R., Lakoma, M. D., Sullivan, A. M., Arnold, R., et al. (2008). A qualitative study of oncologists' approaches to end-of-life care. *Journal of Palliative Medicine, 11,* 893–906.

Jamison, L. (2014). *The Empathy Exams*. London: Granta.

Jeffrey, D. (2016a). Clarifying empathy: The first step to more humane clinical care. *British Journal of General Practice, 66,* 101–102.

Jeffrey, D. (2016b). A duty of kindness. *Journal of the Royal Society of Medicine, 109,* 261–263.

Jeffrey, D. (2016c). Empathy, sympathy and compassion in healthcare: Is there a problem? Is there a difference? Does it matter? *Journal Royal Society Medicine, 109,* 446–452.

Kearney, M. K., Weininger, R. B., Vachon, M. L. S., Harrison, R. L., & Mount, B. M. (2009). Self-care of physicians caring for patients at the end of life "being connected....a key to survival". *JAMA, 301,* 1155–1164.

Kelley, J. M., Kraft-Todd, G., Schapira, L., Kossowsky, J., & Riess, H. (2014). The influence of the patient-clinician relationship on healthcare outcomes: A systematic review and meta-analysis of randomized controlled trials. *PLoS ONE, 9,* e94207.

Kelly, J. (2017). When I say...empathy. *Medical Education, 51,* 573–574.

Kim, S. S., Kaplowitz, S., & Johnston, M. V. (2004). The effects of physician empathy on patient satisfaction and compliance. *Evaluation and the Health Professions, 27,* 237–251.

Kupetz, M. (2014). Empathy displays as interactional achievements—Multimodal and sequential aspects. *Journal of Pragmatics, 61,* 4–34.

Larson, E., & Yao, X. (2005). Clinical empathy as emotional labor in the patient-physician relationship. *JAMA, 293,* 1100–1106.

Light, A., Gupta, T., Burrows, A., Nandakumar, M., Daniel, A., & Karthikeyan, S. (2018). Learning empathy: The medical student perspective. *The Clinical Teacher*. https://doi.org?101111/tct 12801. Accessed December 23, 2018.
Lipps, T. (1903). *Asthetik*. Leipzig, Germany: Leopold Voss Verlag.
Little, P., Everitt, H., Williamson, I., Warner, G., Moore, M., Gould, C., et al. (2001). Preferences of patients for patient centred approach to consultation in primary care: Observational study. *British Medical Journal, 322,* 1–7.
Macintyre, A. (1985). *After Virtue*. London: Duckworth.
Macnaughton, J. (2009). The dangerous practice of empathy. *Lancet, 373,* 1940–1941.
Maguire, P., Faulkner, A., Booth, K., Elliott, C., & Hillier, V. (1996). Helping cancer patients disclose their concerns. *European Journal of Cancer, 32,* 78–81.
Main, A., Walle, E. A., Kho, C., & Halpern, J. (2017). The interpersonal functions of empathy: A relational perspective. *Emotion Review, 9,* 358–366.
Marshall, G. R. E., & Hooker, C. (2016). Empathy and affect: What can empathied bodies do? *Medical Humanities, 42,* 128–134.
Maxwell, B. (2008). *Professional Ethics Education: Studies in Compassionate Empathy*. New York: Springer.
Mercer, S. W., & Reynolds, W. J. (2002). Empathy and quality of care. *British Journal of General Practice, 52,* S9–S12.
Montgomery, K. (2006). *How Doctors Think: Clinical Judgment and the Practice of Medicine*. Oxford: Oxford University Press.
Morse, J. M., Anderson, G., Bottorff, J. L., Yonge, O., O'brien, B., & Solberg, S., et al. (1992). Exploring empathy: A conceptual fit for nursing practice? *Image: The Journal of Nursing Scholarship, 24,* 273–280.
Neumann, M., Scheffer, C., Tauschel, D., Lutz, G., Wirtz, M., & Edelhauser, F. (2012). Physician empathy: Definition, outcome-relevance and its measurement in patient care and medical education. *GMS Zeitschrift fur medizinische Ausbildung, 29,* 1–21.
Neumann, M., Wirtz, M., Bollschweiler, E., Mercer, S., Warm, M., Wolf, J., et al. (2007). Determinants and patient-reported long-term outcomes of physician empathy in oncology: A structural equation modelling approach. *Patient Education and Counseling, 69,* 63–75.
Noddings, N. (1984). *Caring: A Feminine Approach to Ethics and Moral Education*. Berkeley: University of California Press.

Noddings, N. (2013). *Caring: A Relational Approach to Ethics and Moral Education*. Berkeley: University of California Press.
Nogueira-Martins, M. C. F., Nogueira-Martins, L. A., & Turato, E. R. (2006). Medical students' perceptions of their learning about the doctor-patient relationship: A qualitative study. *Medical Education, 40,* 322–328.
Norfolk, T., Birdi, K., & Walsh, D. (2007). The role of empathy in establishing rapport in the consultation: A new model. *Medical Education, 41,* 690–697.
Pedersen, R. (2009). Empirical research on empathy in medicine—A critical review. *Patient Education and Counseling, 76,* 307–322.
Pedersen, R. (2010). Empathy development in medical education—A critical review. *Medical Teacher, 32,* 593–600.
Philips, A., & Taylor, B. (2009). *On Kindness*. London: Hamish Hamilton.
Price, S., Mercer, S., & Macpherson, H. (2006). Practitioner empathy, patient enablement and health outcomes: A prospective study of acupuncture patients. *Patient Education and Counseling, 63,* 239–245.
Rakel, D. P., Hoeft, T. J., Barrett, B. P., Chewning, B. A., Craig, B. M., & Niu, M. (2009). Practitioner empathy and the duration of the common cold. *Family Medicine, 41,* 494–501.
Ratanawongsa, N., Teherani, A., & Hauer, K. E. (2005). Third-year medical students' experiences with dying patients during the internal medicine clerkship: A qualitative study of the informal curriculum. *Academic Medicine, 80,* 641–647.
Riess, H. (2015). The impact of clinical empathy on patients and clinicians: Understanding empathy's side effects. *AJOB Neuroscience, 6,* 51–53.
Rogers, C. (1959). A theory of therapy, personality and interpersonal relationships as developed in the client-centered framework. In S. E. Koch (Ed.), *Psychology: A Study of Science—Formulations of the Person and the Social Context*. New York: McGraw-Hill.
Rogers, C. R. (1961). *On Becoming a Person*. London: Constable.
Roter, D. L., Hall, J. A., Merisca, R., Nordstrom, B., Cretin, D., & Svarstad, B. (1998). Effectiveness of interventions to improve patient compliance: A meta-analysis. *Medical Care, 36,* 1138–1161.
Schutz, A. (1967). *The Phenomenology of the Social World*. Evanston, IL: Northwestern University Press.
Shapiro, J. (2008). Walking a mile in their patients' shoes: Empathy and othering in medical students' education. *Philosophy, Ethics, and Humanities in Medicine, 3,* 10–21.

Slote, M. (2007). *The Ethics of Care and Empathy*. London: Routledge.
Smajdor, A., Stöckl, A., & Salter, C. (2011). The limits of empathy: Problems in medical education and practice. *Journal of Medical Ethics, 37,* 380–383.
Stein, E. (1989). *On the Problem of Empathy (The Collected Works of Edith Stein Vol. 3)*. Washington, DC: ICS Publishers.
Stepien, K. A., & Baernstein, A. (2006). Educating for empathy—A review. *Journal of General Internal Medicine, 21,* 524–530.
Stocks, E. L., Lishner, D., & Decker, S. K. (2009). Altruism or psychological escape: Why does empathy promote prosocial behavior? *European Journal of Social Psychology, 39,* 649–665.
Stueber, K. (2006). *Rediscovering Empathy: Agency, Folk Psychology and the Human Sciences*. Cambridge: MIT Press.
Suchman, A. L., Markakis, K., Beckman, H. B., & Frankel, R. (1997). A model of empathic communication in the medical interview. *JAMA, 277,* 678–682.
Sulzer, S. H., Feinstein, N. W., & Wendland, C. L. (2016). Assessing empathy development in medical education: A systematic review. *Medical Education, 50,* 300–310.
Svenaeus, F. (2014). Empathy as a necessary condition of phronesis: A line of thought for medical ethics. *Medicine, Health Care and Philosophy, 17,* 293–299.
Svenaeus, F. (2015). The relationship between empathy and sympathy in good health care. *Medicine, Health Care and Philosophy, 18,* 267–277.
Tavakol, S., Dennick, R., & Tavakol, M. (2012). Medical students' understanding of empathy: A phenomenological study. *Medical Education, 46,* 306–316.
Tichner, E. (1909). *Lectures on the Experimental Psychology of the Thought Processes*. New York: Macmillan.
Vagle, M. D. (2016). *Crafting Phenomenological Research*. London: Routledge.
Von Dietze, E., & Orb, A. (2000). Compassionate care: A moral dimension of nursing. *Nursing Inquiry, 7,* 166–174.
Warmington, S. (2012). Practising engagement: Infusing communication with empathy and compassion in medical students' clinical encounters. *Health, 16,* 327–342.
Watson, J., & Greenburg, L. (2011). Empathic resonance: A neuroscience perspective. In J. E. Decety & W. Ickes (Eds.), *The Social Neuroscience of Empathy*. London: MIT Press.

Wensing, M., Jung, H. P., Mainz, J., Olesen, F., & Grol, R. (1998). A systematic review of the literature on patient priorities for general practice care. Part 1: Description of the research domain. *Social Science and Medicine, 47,* 1573–1588.

Wispé, L. (1986). The distinction between sympathy and empathy: To call forth a concept, a word is needed. *Journal of Personality and Social Psychology, 50,* 314.

Zaki, J., & Williams, W. C. (2013). Interpersonal emotion regulation. *Emotion, 13,* 803.

4

Emotions and Empathy

Overview

Three themes emerged from the students' stories relating to emotional aspects of empathy: the risks of emotional connection with patients, professional detachment and emotional regulation. In this chapter, students describe their reservations about sharing emotions with a patient—the risk to themselves of becoming stressed and the harmful influence of emotions on clinical decision-making. They also reflect on the potential benefits of emotional connection with patients. The students described how they were taught to distance themselves from patients and so came to see this as being 'professional'. The case for this 'detached concern' is explored and the risks and benefits of detachment as a coping strategy are debated. The students described the way in which they strike a balance between connection and detachment. Appropriate boundary setting is discussed and the importance of self-awareness, reflective practice and student support is stressed.

D. I. Jeffrey, *Exploring Empathy with Medical Students*,
https://doi.org/10.1007/978-3-030-11211-0_4

Risks and Benefits of Emotional Connection with a Patient

The Risks of Emotional Connection

While most students maintained that sharing emotions was an integral part of empathy, they also expressed concerns about the risks of this connection. These concerns related to two areas: that they might become overwhelmed by emotions, or that emotions might cloud objective clinical decision-making. Fiona saw a danger in becoming too emotional and suggested a need to develop mechanisms to cope with the emotions she encountered in practice.

> it could be potentially very bad for an individual to take on all that emotion and therefore generally develop coping mechanisms to deal with dealing with all these sort of emotional luggage that comes with it. (Fiona, Year 3)

There was uncertainty amongst the students about the effect of emotions on clinical decision-making. While acknowledging the risks of being too emotionally involved, Fiona valued experiencing the feelings of the patient in clinical decision-making.

> the patient's emotions always have to be taken into account in your decision making but I feel you feeling them yourself doesn't, you don't need to. But I think you got to be able to. I don't really think you can understand emotions without feeling them. (Fiona, Year 2)

On the other hand, Marilyn was clear in her view that emotions may cloud judgement or even harm the doctor or the patient. She cited the general prohibition on doctors treating their own family as evidence for the need to avoid emotions in decision-making.

> it will cloud your judgment and it might not make you as good a physician. (Marilyn, Year 2)

Some students were concerned that by getting too involved with the patient they risked projecting their own feelings onto the patient.

> I think it is almost if you have too much empathy you may occasionally try to start to make decisions for the other people because you feel you understand them so much, when it is still their decision. (Bill, Year 1)

Neville claimed that there was a widespread belief amongst medical students and doctors that emotions threatened objectivity. He rejected this belief, affirming that emotions should be taken into consideration in clinical decision-making.

> I think the biggest reason is because it interferes with their thought process of being objective and being evidence based. (Neville, Year 4)

> but unless you understand what the patient wants you can't do anything for them, any therapeutic intervention. (Neville, Year 5)

Students may respond to their perceived risks of emotional connection by distancing themselves from patients and by restricting their empathy to cognitive rather than affective domains. However, the majority of students argued that sharing feelings was necessary for empathy, although some were less certain. One student claimed that a doctor should not share emotions with a patient, maintaining that she would rather be treated by a competent, brusque surgeon than a kindly less competent one. She was employing a reductive argument, perpetuating a binary perspective of empathy. McNaughton pointed out that such dichotomies merely fostered the marginalisation of emotion in professionalism and practice (McNaughton 2013). In the medical literature, emotional empathy is usually considered from the perspective of the patient. However, some students considered that it was appropriate to show patients that they were affected by emotion (Håkansson and Montgomery 2003). This was further evidence that they did not favour a detached construction of empathy (Marshall and Hooker 2016).

The relegation of emotions as unsafe in clinical training has contributed to a lack of study of the humanities in medical education and so further diminished their visibility in training (McNaughton 2013). In this medical school, there was little formal input of the humanities in the curriculum, other than a single self-selected module available to a few students. Although emotional sharing in empathy was regarded by some authors as essential to empathising, the dominant message the students received was that detachment and objectivity were more appropriate (Greenson 1960; Halpern 2001; Gillies and Sheehan 2005). McNaughton asked a pertinent question, 'Where has the idea originated that to be a good doctor one must remove emotion from reason, or so dilute it for the patient's benefit, to result in detached concern?' (McNaughton 2013; Halpern 2001). Patients also appeared to want their doctors to demonstrate empathetic concern (Mercer and Reynolds 2002). Broyard (1992) described his experience as a patient, saying of his doctor:

> To the typical physician, my illness is a routine incident in his rounds, while for me it's the crisis of my life. I would feel better if I had a doctor who at least perceived this incongruity. (Broyard 1992, p. 45).

Most students maintained that true empathy required not only understanding the patient's emotion but experiencing it to some degree. Some students reflected that an emotional understanding was necessary for clinical judgement and to develop a healing relationship. Some refined this view by describing experiencing as having a 'taste' of the patient's emotion rather than taking on the full force of their suffering. In this way, they were aware of the quality of the patient's emotion without its potentially overwhelming intensity. Agosta (2014) supported this view by claiming that in empathy, the student took a sample of the suffering of the patient without over-identifying with the other person. Decety and Lamm (2011) maintained that empathic concern inevitably resulted in a sharing of emotion, in that the student felt the pain of the patient, while remaining aware that it was the other's pain.

The literature supported the students' views that emotionally engaged doctors communicated more effectively with patients. Consequently, patients were more engaged with treatment decisions (Halpern 2014; Girgis and Sanson-Fisher 1995; Kim et al. 2004; Kozlowski et al. 2017).

It appeared from the students' conversations that empathy began with being open to becoming affected by the patient's emotions (Marshall and Hooker 2016; Clark 2010). Gillies and Sheehan (2005) suggested that emotions enabled a doctor to focus on his or her work and were not primitive forces, but should be used by the doctor to guide her responses in a particular context. Empathy, by most of the students' descriptions, seemed to reflect Buber's I–Thou relationship rather than the objectifying I–It relationship and so involved them in experiencing some of the patient's suffering (Buber 2004).

While most students said that they wanted to connect with patients emotionally, some expressed concerns that engaging with emotions might lead to stress and burnout and so affect their 'objective' clinical judgement. At the heart of this debate was the need to clarify the difference between appropriate empathetic concern and personal distress which may result from over-identifying with the patient (Decety and Lamm 2011). There is evidence from the neurosciences, sociology and psychology that that cognition is connected to emotions which contribute to decision-making (Immordino-Yang and Damasio 2007; McNaughton 2013; Kozlowski et al. 2017). However, the idea that emotions are disruptive, and need to be controlled, is deeply ingrained in medical education and practice (Montgomery 2006). Heyhoe et al. (2016) recently reviewed how emotions contributed to clinical decisions and concluded that they played an integral part in patient safety. Halpern (2001) has argued for a form of professional empathy which included emotional-based reasoning (Ekman and Halpern 2015). Other authors have also argued for the role of emotions in clinical decision-making (Decety and Fotopoulou 2014; Isen et al. 1991; Kozlowski et al. 2017). Damasio commenting on the intrinsic role of emotions in decision-making argued that the universality of emotions in human beings implied that this innate ability enabled us to relate to each other at deeper levels of understanding (Damasio 1999). Salovey et al. argued that emotions are the primary sources of motivations to act and they provide the individual with information which affects their decisions (Salovey et al. 2008). Furthermore, Irving and Dickson (2004) argued that decreasing distancing, either as physical space or as psychological involvement, tended to increase the level of perceived empathy.

While some students observed doctors using detachment as a coping strategy, many claimed that they would feel stressed and unfulfilled if they were compelled to work in such a way. These views concurred with research which suggested that empathetic doctors had more job satisfaction and less burnout than colleagues who coped by detachment from patients (Kearney et al. 2009; Zenasni et al. 2012). It seemed from the literature that even if doctors tried to suppress their feelings by distancing themselves from patients, they could not avoid having emotional attitudes towards patients (Larson and Yao 2005). Agosta (2014) argued that without empathic understanding students experienced burnout. He claimed that without affective empathy they behaved with detached concern, in which case they were at risk of drawing the wrong conclusions about the patient's experience (Agosta 2014). He further argued that in using detached concern, the patient became an association of symptoms, rather than a struggling human being worthy of respect (Agosta 2014). Charon suggested that narrative medicine has highlighted the importance of engagement with the patient which included an ability to be moved by the patient (Charon 2001).

Sharing Vulnerability

The students maintained that they wanted to share vulnerability with patients in the process of empathising. Krznaric emphasised that empathy inevitably exposed our vulnerability and involved sharing part of oneself with others (Krznaric 2014). Some students suggested that self-disclosure of their own experiences of illness could be helpful in establishing empathy. However, one student reflected that, in the clinical years, she had become wary of sharing details of her own illness. In some sense, this self-disclosure was an essential part of the relational aspect of empathy in that the empathetic student sensed when such self-disclosure was appropriate (Gelhaus 2012). Although the personal experience of suffering may have informed the student's empathy, it should not be assumed that the patient necessarily shared the same feelings.

Ricoeur explored the connection between vulnerability and empathy. He argued that although there are differences between people, we are bound together in a search for mutual recognition and understanding (Ricoeur 1992). He claimed that we are simultaneously capable and vulnerable, blurring role boundaries that assigned competence to doctors and vulnerability to patients. He further asserted that selfhood and otherness cannot be separated, that to be able to see oneself as another implied being able to see another as oneself, so the suffering of others becomes our suffering (Ricoeur 1992). His philosophy challenges scientific objectivity in offering an ethics of imperfection which fosters empathy.

Detached Concern

Students talked about neglecting emotional connection with the patient and restricting empathy to the cognitive domain, where they became distant from the patient. They expressed concerns that such distancing could cause stress. Olive feared that although connecting emotionally could lead to burnout, too much distancing could lead to ineffective patient care.

> I don't think it leads to effective doctoring really, if you try and distance yourself too much. (Olive, Year 1)

Fiona was concerned that if a doctor was detached, there was a risk that the patient would not disclose their real concerns. Paula did not think detachment was appropriate, implying that doctors should be motivated towards working closely with patients.

> if they[patients]don't feel like they are being listened to or understood then they will stop bothering to give the information. (Fiona, Year 1)

> doesn't seem very healthy to be entirely detached from patients […] I think it would be wrong to be entirely detached from all the patients. (Paula, Year 3)

Students shared their reservations as to how effective such detachment would be as a coping mechanism, inferring that detachment could lead to its own stresses.

> no matter how much you try to distance yourself there must be something will upset you and resonate with you on an individual level. (Olive, Year 1)

Kim questioned whether detached doctors found it more stressful to avoid exploring feelings, speculating whether their detachment was due to external factors or to the doctor's personality. Lisa reflected that if she had to work in a detached way, she would feel unfulfilled and guilty. Some students noticed that doctors from certain specialities were more likely than others to exhibit detachment from their patients.

> maybe the people that don't explore those type of things don't find it stressful to not explore that but [...] what causes them not to go into it in the first place,? Whether it is [a] time constraint or an innate issue? (Kim, Year 4)

> I probably feel that I could have done more. I hadn't quite completely fulfilled what I really should have been doing that day. (Lisa, Year 4)

> surgeons, I suppose, would find it easier not to think too much about the patient under the covers. (Olive, Year 1)

Some students suggested that perhaps older patients might prefer doctors to be more detached but considered that the majority of patients preferred doctors who connected with them.

> older generations expect a doctor to be like that and possibly strange or unnerving if they were not like that, they might not trust you, but most but with most patients they prefer to connect. (Bill, Year 1)

> the patients didn't really appreciate the people who were very detached. (Fiona, Year 1)

The students debated the reasons why a doctor would behave in a detached manner. Jenny suggested that a detached doctor might save time as patients may be reluctant to approach them.

> if you look very disinterested and engaged in your environment people are more likely to leave you. (Jenny, Year 1)

Kim suggested a number of reasons for doctors employing distancing tactics: their personality, workload, time pressures and a medical culture of immunity to feelings. There was a risk that in such a culture of routines, targets and guidelines, doctors might forget that every patient was an individual.

> I suppose another part of it an immunity in a way you have done it so many times, it is so routine you forget that every patient is a new patient. (Kim, Year 4)

Another reason Kim suggested that doctors distanced themselves was as a form of self-protection from emotional distress. Helen did not think that remaining cold and detached was best for the patient and questioned who was benefitting by being detached.

> I think it is self-protective [...] it is definitely easier not to take on the patient's problems, not explore what they are feeling. (Kim, Year 4)

> I think there is a tricky balance somewhere on there because I don't think it is safer to stay cold and distant I think it detrimental to the patient to stay cold and distant. (Helen, Year 1)

Paula argued that in some situations, it may not be necessary to explore the patient's feelings—cognitive empathy alone might be appropriate. Marilyn implied that there was a balance to be achieved in effective empathy.

> maybe there is an argument for patients who are presenting with something that is quick and simply to fix and you can just maybe don't need to go any more than that. (Paula, Year 6)

> You have to have some kind of distance but there is a big difference between that and not caring at all. (Marilyn, Year 1)

Students often linked detachment with medical professionalism. In a 'detached concern', or cognitive, model of empathising, understanding is situated within the student rather than the patient (Halpern 2001). They perceived that professionalism was taught as being detached from patients. They received conflicting messages from the medical school, an overt message to connect with patients, and yet in practice they observed doctors who remained detached from the patient's emotional concerns.

> one of the things you hear all the time is that doctors should have a professional detachment. (Edward, Year 1)

> we get lectures on professionalism and it is always is[...]keep a safe distance. (Helen, Year 2)

> I think the way we are taught to be professional does not account for necessarily always being empathetic. (Paula, Year 4)

The students argued that maintaining a professional distance was inappropriate. Some students suggested that being warm and empathetic was compatible with professionalism. Sometimes professionalism was viewed as a form of stoicism, a cold, emotional detachment.

> professionals definitely need to have compassion they need to be warm and friendly people to a certain extent and there is a boundary where that becomes unprofessional. I think there is a spectrum of behaviours where things can become unprofessional. I think some doctors can be very stoic I think that would not necessarily be perceived as unprofessional by a lot of patients. (Connie, Year 1)

> I think there might be a misconception amongst people that if you have to be professional you have got not be emotional, not show that side of yourself to patients. (Neville, Year 4)

Marilyn was also critical of the call to be professional and emphasised the importance of context in relation to empathy. While Diana implied professionalism numbed her emotions, Paula considered that professionalism was inadequately addressed in the curriculum.

> there are going to be patients that strike a chord with me and 'Is it professional?'. Pfft professional, professional. They are keen on us all being so damn professional. There are some patients who will appreciate that and

> there are some patients who need you to be strong for them. It depends on the patient. (Marilyn, Year 2)

> I think sometimes professionalism numbs, numbs human emotional function. (Diane, Year 6)

> [on]occasions throw in something about professionalism but it is more so kind of an assignments or it is not a huge thing. (Paula, Year 4)

Gina suggested that there was an unrealistic standard of medical professionalism expected of students.

> the way they talk about professionalism is almost like you are under scrutiny to be this sort of sub-perfect human being. (Gina, Year 6)

Previous studies showed that students described situations where showing feelings was discouraged by senior doctors, with the result that students became reluctant to show emotions (Eikeland et al. 2014). Instead, students linked their need to be professional with detachment from patients (Tavakol et al. 2012).

Professional Distance

Medical professionalism has, like empathy, been defined in different ways, for example,

> a set of values, behaviours, and relationships that underpins the trust the public has in doctors. (Working Party of the Royal College of Physicians 2005)

The Royal College of Physicians Report proposed that doctors were committed to integrity, compassion, altruism, continuous improvement, excellence and working in partnership with members of the wider healthcare team (Working Party of the Royal College of Physicians 2005). The GMC also listed the duties of a doctor in Good Medical Practice (General Medical Council 2013).

It is paradoxical that while descriptions of professionalism include humanistic values such as empathy, students gain an impression of professionalism as distancing from patients (West and Shanafelt 2007). The debate in the literature around medical professionalism mirrors much of that surrounding empathy: a lack of definition and uncertainty as to whether it can be taught or assessed (Levenson et al. 2008; Rogers and Ballantyne 2010; Cruess et al. 2014). Perhaps the issue of the patient's trust in the doctor lies at the heart of both empathy and professionalism. Empathy is thought to engender trust, while professionalism is predicated on a need to establish public trust in doctors (Hafferty and Castellani 2011).

Doctors have acquired professional identities, so that they come to think, act and feel like a physician, since at least the time of Hippocrates (Cruess et al. 2014). However, it is only recently that studies have analysed the nature of this identity. Some authors describe 'nostalgic professionalism' which emphasises the altruistic role of the individual physician (Cruess et al. 2014). They have also argued for a professional identity which embraced teamwork (Cruess et al. 2014). However, 'nostalgic professionalism' might be incorporated into a more humane form of a virtue-based professionalism.

The professed values of the medical school creating compassionate doctors did not resonate with the students' experiences of professionalism as distancing from the patient. Ekman and Krasner (2016) claimed that a culture of empathy aversion in medical education had generated a professional stance of 'detached concern', which neglected the emotional experience of the patient. Despite the GMC requiring students and doctors to be both caring and competent, it appeared that medical professionalism continued to imply emotional detachment (General Medical Council 2013; Kerasidou and Horn 2016; Hilton and Southgate 2007).

Many years ago, Osler claimed that by excluding emotions doctors gained a special objective insight into the patient's suffering. He implied that empathy could be achieved through detachment (Osler 1963). One consequence of adopting 'detached concern' as a model for medical professionalism is that the emotions of a doctor or patient may be perceived as a threat to the supposed need for objectivity and a risk to patient safety (Kerasidou and Horn 2016; Hegazi and Wilson 2013;

Coulehan 1995). There is now an accepted view that doctors should respond to the suffering of patients with objectivity and detachment (Montgomery 2006). However, the prevailing view is challenged in this book and by several authors (Halpern 2001; Shapiro 2011; Spiro et al. 1993; Coulehan 2005). Halpern described how the model of detached concern prevailed in the medical culture despite the fact that there was little evidence that establishing an emotional connection with a patient led to a negative outcome (Halpern 2001). I suggest that detachment is not necessary for sound medical judgement because emotional insights can and should inform clinical decision-making (Coulehan 1995; Mayer et al. 2008; Halpern 2001; Kozlowski et al. 2017).

It is relevant to question why some students adopted distancing tactics such as detached concern (Jones 2010). Brody (1997) argued that if doctors were detached, the patient's suffering remained without meaning and healing was impeded. Detachment may be adopted as a mechanism to prevent burnout and remain composed when faced with emotionally challenging situations (Kerasidou and Horn 2016). Although studies have suggested that even if doctors try to suppress their feelings, they must have emotional attitudes towards patients (Halpern 2007). Students became aware of a divergence between those who continue to strive for academic recognition where others concentrated on meeting the needs of the patient. An emphasis on objectivity may lead students to strive towards competence in practice, neglecting a humanistic approach (Allen et al. 2008; Cribb and Bignold 1999; Evans et al. 1993; Coulehan and Williams 2001).

Another risk of promoting empathy as a kind of detached concern is that empathy may continue to be seen as a set of cognitive skills rather than as a virtue of a good doctor (Shapiro 2012; Winefield and Chur-Hansen 2000). There is also a risk that if empathy is viewed as a performance rather than a deeply held commitment, it could become selective and restricted to likeable patients (Shapiro 2012). Authors have described the relationship between a doctor and patient as essentially an emotional connection (Coulehan 1995, 2009; Bub 2007). A detached form of practice may deprive doctors of emotional fulfilment in their practice and could become an inbuilt attitude which eventually spreads into their personal life (Montgomery 2006).

Balancing Connection and Detachment—The Self-Other Boundary

Students were concerned to achieve an appropriate balance to meet the patient's needs and yet not to become overwhelmed. They reflected on how regulating distressing emotions were an integral part of a doctor's role.

> you have to be empathetic to do medicine[...]but not too empathetic. (Paula, Year 5)

> you need to keep your empathy in check but that doesn't mean that you can't have any, but you need some control over it. You need some level of distance. (Marilyn, Year 2)

The students admitted that many found achieving this balance was difficult, particularly if they had a personal experience of the patient's illness or were stressed.

> I think part of the challenge of medicine is not to take these things to heart, you have to kind of be able put them aside a little bit and draw lines. But I think sometimes that is really, really difficult to do. (Kim, Year 6)

> if there is something that is very personal, like you have had a personal experience of it is more difficult to maybe maintain that distance. (Kim, Year 6)

The students viewed detachment as inappropriate yet appreciated that in order to have an emotional connection with patients there needed to be a mechanism to regulate their empathy: a self-other boundary.

The students described a satisfactory empathetic approach as one where an appropriate psychological boundary existed between themselves and the patient. This was not to distance themselves but to recognise where the self ends and where the other person's problems are situated.

> you have to learn from the patient and learn from what they felt but progress through [the] medical and not get bogged down in every patient's emotion. (Kim, Year 4)

They discussed practical ways of developing this self-other boundary: compartments, patient experience, reflection, curiosity, resilience and support.

Compartments

Marilyn described a process of 'compartmentalisation', which did not mean complete detachment from emotions, but acknowledged a degree of distance. Fiona explained that 'compartmentalisation' included ways of achieving a balance between work and her personal life.

> there are detached doctors but I think they are terrible. I think more compartmentalisation is important. (Marilyn, Year 1)

> Leave work at work and then you have your home and your family and friends and people to support you and I think that is compartments. (Fiona, Year 3)

Patient Experience

Some students suggested that the setting of boundaries between detachment and connection came with clinical experience. Olive compared the skill of empathising with learning to drive, suggesting that the self-other boundary became instinctive with experience.

> I think as you go through your training and you build and meet more and more patients and deal with more of these situations you build that how, what works best. (Fiona, Year 3)

> It is just like if you are driving, you have to think about every single action you are doing, I am changing gears de de de and suddenly you have been driving a few years and doesn't require so much thinking. (Olive, Year 3)

Reflection

Students described the importance of reflecting on experiences as part of the process of setting a self-other boundary. Creating a self-other boundary involved both greater self-awareness and a natural sense of the other person as being distinct from oneself. This process involved developing mechanisms of emotional control which required effort at first, but later became a natural response.

> Being empathetic in the long term is being able to pause and reflect and appreciate the circumstances of someone other than yourself. It breeds resilience and I think it is something that comes as you mature and [...] it is dynamic and [...] your own perception of empathy changes as you get older and as you see things. (Gina, Year 6)

Curiosity

Students suggested that taking an interest in patients, in a form of clinical curiosity, was another mechanism of maintaining the self-other boundary.

> you have to have professional boundaries but that doesn't mean you can't attempt to really explore what a patient sees. (Gina, Year 6)

> it is a little a distance but it is a perspective of the other person. You are not completely immersed in it. (Neville, Year 6)

Resilience

A few students talked about empathy and resilience in relation to an appropriate self-other boundary. Some saw resilience as being empathetic without burdening oneself with emotions, linking it with detached concern.

> I think that is part of resilience is to be able to be empathetic without burdening yourself with everything. (Fiona, Year 2)

Gina argued that resilience was a 'bandwagon' that medical educators were jumping on at present. She implied that there was a risk of equating resilience with distancing from the patient's emotional distress.

> resilience is one of the words they throw about when talk about coping with life as a doctor. (Gina, Year 6)

> you need to build up a certain level of tolerance where everything you see doesn't shake you which I guess is almost kind of almost putting up a wall and stepping back. (Gina, Year 6)

Support

The students talked about how stress could reduce their empathy and their need for support. Helen implied that taking on the problems of others can be overwhelming and there was a need for support as a part of regulating their empathy.

> in order to be able to empathise you have to an extent take on someone's problems [...]you can't do that endlessly and relentlessly every day without somebody doing it for you. (Helen, Year 3)

Emotional Regulation: Balancing Connection and Detachment

Central to this research has been finding that the students struggled to achieve an appropriate balance between detachment from and connection with a patient. They discussed how to create a psychological self-other boundary and so to find an appropriate balance.

Emotional regulation is the ability to modify one's emotional experiences and responses in context (Shapiro 2013; Gross and Thompson 2007). The students claimed that they lacked guidance on how to regulate their emotions, so risked being emotionally overwhelmed in connecting with patients. In a study by Meitar et al. (2009), students who expressed their emotions and addressed the emotions expressed by the patient were most likely to demonstrate empathy. Shapiro maintained that in the absence of appropriate support, about managing emotions, students might resort to distancing from patients (Shapiro 2008). She suggested a paradigm that helps students to develop a tolerance for imperfection in themselves and others, an acceptance of shared emotional vulnerability and which values the existence of difference (Shapiro 2008). Halpern (2001) suggested that empathy was therapeutic because it relied on a doctors' ability to understand the patient's emotional point of view rather than having intense positive feelings towards the patient (Halpern 2001). In empathy, she claimed, one was emotionally engaged with the other and at the same time was able to reflect on the emotions, knowing that they originated in the other person (Halpern 2001).

Resilience was described as one mechanism for achieving a balance but the students were concerned that it might lead to detachment. They also suggested that achieving an appropriate self-other boundary might come with clinical experience and greater self-awareness. The self-other boundary was explored by Frank (2004), who described the idea of alterity and its relationship to dialogue. Alterity involved the recognition of the other person as being separate from oneself and allowed the possibility of genuine dialogue and true empathy (Warmington 2012). In an empathetic encounter, both the student and the patient were enabled to have a voice, and in so doing, their alterity was respected (Frank 2004). Bondi (2014) developed these ideas by claiming that there should be an ongoing sense of the alterity of the other. She suggested that this was an unconscious process in which the student was both a subjectively engaged participant in a two-person relationship and also an observer of that relationship. This process allowed the student to be subjectively absorbed in the patient's narrative as well as maintaining a capacity to step back and reflect on that absorption (Bondi 2014).

The students described how in spite of being aware of the dangers of personal distress in taking a self-orientated perspective, they sometimes had an initial thought of 'What might this be like for me?' (Batson 2011). This thought was followed by a more considered, other-orientated perspective, 'What is this like for the patient?' Taking an other-orientated perspective was claimed to be part of forming a psychological boundary with the other person and was thought to be an essential part of empathising. These views resonate with the work of Rogers (1961), who claimed that although empathy should involve a deep engagement with the patient, it did not mean that the student lost sight of where the self ends and the other begins. He stressed that empathy involved entering the perceived world of the other person 'as if' one were the other person, but without ever losing the 'as if' condition (Rogers 1959). Bondi (2008) also described a self-other boundary which resonates with this view. In true empathy, the student was emotionally engaged with the patient, and at the same time, she was able to reflect on these emotions, knowing that they originated in the other person (Halpern 2001). In retaining a sense of the self-other boundary, empathy differed from identification which can result in personal distress and burnout (Decety and Ickes 2011).

Agosta (2014) approached the problem of emotional regulation from a Heideggerian perspective by adopting a broad sense of empathising which he claimed was a powerful resource against suffering and burnout. He argued that if a student was overwhelmed and experienced burnout from engagement with the patient's suffering, then she was not using empathy properly. He suggested that in this situation the student should recalibrate their empathy. This was reflected in the students' descriptions of adjusting their level of empathy to meet the patient's needs. Conversely, if the students found that they were behaving in a detached way, Agosta suggested that they needed to increase their empathetic receptivity (Agosta 2014). Indeed, a student described a 'massive wake-up call' when she realised how medicalised she had become in her interactions with patients. Agosta (2014) described the boundary between self and the other as a permeable boundary, able to be crossed by emotions and experience.

To maintain the delicate psychological balance between detachment and connection, the students described their need to be self-aware, to reflect on their work and to have access to support (Balint 1957; Bondi 2014). Students described how they were less empathetic when stressed and how much they needed and appreciated support. Marshall and Hooker (2016) suggested that stress may inhibit emotional engagement and that conversely support, which reduces stress, allowed students to be more open to emotions.

Some studies suggest that students struggle to empathise because they did not know how to regulate their emotions (Eikeland et al. 2014; Ratanawongsa et al. 2005). Many students wanted to be both competent and empathetic but were uncertain how to balance an emotional connection with the patient with detachment in their clinical decision-making (Eikeland et al. 2014). Students suggested that a little distance from the patient's emotions might be appropriate but too much might lead to apparent indifference (Ratanawongsa et al. 2005; Eikeland et al. 2014). They were concerned that detachment implied that they did not engage in a genuine dialogue with the patient (Eikeland et al. 2014).

There is little discussion in the wider medical education literature about how students might manage their emotions (Meier et al. 2001; Coulehan 1995). Shapiro suggested that medical education promotes professional alexithymia, a term used to describe people who have difficulty recognising, processing and regulating emotions (Shapiro 2011). One possible result of such a learning environment is that medical students may deny their emotions (Jennings 2009).

The fundamental ambivalence of empathy is the risk it exposes to the students when sharing their vulnerability and emotions with others; so there is a need to find a balance between empathy and detachment (Ballatt and Campling 2011). If students are to empathise, they must connect with patients in this uneasy state, but to do so they need the support and guidance of experienced doctors (Ballatt and Campling 2011; Bleakley and Bligh 2008).

It seemed from the students' stories that there was a lack of understanding of the distinction between appropriate empathetic concern and harmful personal distress (Decety and Meyer 2008). An empathetic response results if an affective emotional resonance between the student and patient is combined with cognitive reflection and the maintenance of an appropriate self-other boundary. However, if a self-orientated perspective is taken by the student, the result is personal distress and distancing from the patient (Ekman and Halpern 2015).

Key Points

- Detached concern persists as the model for medical professionalism.
- Students wanted to connect emotionally with patients rather than distancing themselves.
- Students felt that emotions should play a part in clinical decision-making.
- Students claimed that they lacked guidance on emotional regulation.

References

Agosta, L. (2014). A rumor of empathy: Reconstructing Heidegger's contribution to empathy and empathic clinical practice. *Medicine, Health Care and Philosophy, 17*(2), 281–292.

Allen, D., Wainwright, M., Mount, B., & Hutchinson, T. (2008). The wounding path to becoming healers: Medical students' apprenticeship experiences. *Medical Teacher, 30*(3), 260–264.

Balint, M. (1957). *The Doctor His Patient and the Illness*. London: Tavistock.

Ballatt, J., & Campling, P. (2011). *Intelligent Kindness*. London: RCPsych.

Batson, C. (2011). These things called empathy: Eight related but distinct phenomena. In J. Decety & W. Ickes (Eds.), *The Social Neuroscience of Empathy*. Cambridge: MIT Press.

Bleakley, A., & Bligh, J. (2008). Students learning from patients: Let's get real in medical education. *Advances in Health Sciences Education, 13*(1), 89–107.

Bondi, L. (2008). On the relational dynamics of caring: A psychotherapeutic approach to emotional and power dimensions of women's care work. *Gender, Place and Culture, 15*(3), 249–265.

Bondi, L. (2014). Understanding feelings: Engaging with unconscious communication and embodied knowledge. *Emotion, Space and Society, 10*, 44–54.

Brody, H. (1997). Who gets to tell the story? Narrative in postmodern bioethics. In H. Nelson (Ed.), *Stories and Their Limits: Narrative Approaches to Bioethics*. London: Routledge.

Broyard, A. (1992). *Intoxicated by My Illness: And Other Writings on Life and Death*. New York: Fawcett Columbine.

Bub, B. (2007). Focusing and the healing sequence: Reclaiming authentic emotions as an aid to communication and well-being in medicine. *Explore: The Journal of Science and Healing, 3*(4), 413–416.

Buber, M. (2004). *I and Thou*. London: Continuum.

Charon, R. (2001). Narrative medicine—A model for empathy, reflection, profession, and trust. *JAMA, 286*(15), 1897–1902.

Clark, A. J. (2010). Empathy: An integral model in the counseling process. *Journal of Counseling & Development, 88*(3), 348–356.

Coulehan, J. (2005). Today's professionalism: Engaging the mind but not the heart. *Academic Medicine, 80*(10), 892–898.

Coulehan, J. (2009). Compassionate solidarity: Suffering, poetry, and medicine. *Perspectives in Biology and Medicine, 52*(4), 585–603.

Coulehan, J., & Williams, P. C. (2001). Vanquishing virtue: The impact of medical education. *Academic Medicine, 76*(6), 598–605.

Coulehan, J. L. (1995). Tenderness and steadiness: Emotions in medical practice. *Literature and Medicine, 14*(2), 222–236.

Cribb, A., & Bignold, S. (1999). Towards the reflexive medical school: The hidden curriculum and medical education research. *Studies in Higher Education, 24*(2), 195–209.

Cruess, R. L., Cruess, S. R., Boudreau, J. D., Snell, L., & Steinert, Y. (2014). Reframing medical education to support professional identity formation. *Academic Medicine, 89*(11), 1446–1451.

Damasio, A. R. (1999). *The Feeling of What Happens: Body and Emotion in the Making of Consciousness*. London: Vintage.

Decety, J., & Fotopoulou, A. (2014). Why empathy has a beneficial impact on others in medicine: Unifying theories. *Frontiers in Behavioral Neuroscience, 8*, 1–11.

Decety, J., & Ickes, W. (2011). *The Social Neuroscience of Empathy*. Cambridge: MIT Press.

Decety, J., & Lamm, C. (2011). Empathy versus personal distress: Recent evidence from social neuroscience. In J. Decety & W. Ickes (Eds.), *The Social Neuroscience of Empathy*. Cambridge: MIT Press.

Decety, J., & Meyer, M. (2008). From emotion resonance to empathic understanding: A social developmental neuroscience account. *Development and Psychopathology, 20*(4), 1053–1080.

Eikeland, H. L., Ornes, K., Finset, A., & Pedersen, R. (2014). The physician's role and empathy—A qualitative study of third year medical students. *BMC Medical Education, 14*(1), 165–173.

Ekman, E., & Halpern, J. (2015). Professional distress and meaning in health care: Why professional empathy can help. *Social Work in Health Care, 54*(7), 633–650.

Ekman, E., & Krasner, M. (2016). Empathy in medicine: Neuroscience, education and challenges. *Medical Teacher, 39*(2), 164–173.

Evans, B., Stanley, R., & Burrows, G. (1993). Measuring medical students' empathy skills. *British Journal of Medical Psychology, 66*(2), 121–133.

Frank, A. (2004). *The Renewal of Generosity*. Chicago: University of Chicago Press.

Gelhaus, P. (2012). The desired moral attitude of the physician: (I) Empathy. *Medicine, Health Care and Philosophy, 15*(2), 103–113.

General Medical Council. (2013). *Good Medical Practice*. London: General Medical Council.

Gillies, J., & Sheehan, M. (2005). Perceptual capacity and the good GP: Invisible, yet indispensable for quality of care. *British Journal of General Practice, 55*(521), 974–977.

Girgis, A., & Sanson-Fisher, R. W. (1995). Breaking bad news: Consensus guidelines for medical practitioners. *Journal of Clinical Oncology, 13*(9), 2449–2456.

Greenson, R. (1960). Empathy and its vicissitudes. *The International Journal of Psycho-Analysis, 41*, 418.

Gross, J. J., & Thompson, R. A. (2007). Emotion regulation: Conceptual foundations. In J. Gross (Ed.), *Handbook of Emotion Regulation*. New York: Guilford Press.

Hafferty, F. W., & Castellani, B. (2011). Two cultures: Two ships—The rise of a professionalism movement within modern medicine and medical sociology's disappearance from the professionalism debate. In B. Pescosolido (Ed.), *Handbook of the Sociology of Health, Illness, and Healing: A Blueprint for the 21st Century.* New York: Springer.

Håkansson, J., & Montgomery, H. (2003). Empathy as an interpersonal phenomenon. *Journal of Social and Personal Relationships, 20*(3), 267–284.

Halpern, J. (2001). *From Detached Concern to Empathy: Humanizing Medical Practice*. Oxford: Oxford University Press.

Halpern, J. (2007). Empathy and patient–physician conflicts. *Journal of General Internal Medicine, 22*(5), 696–700.

Halpern, J. (2014). From idealized clinical empathy to empathic communication in medical care. *Medicine, Health Care and Philosophy, 17*(2), 301–311.

Hegazi, I., & Wilson, I. (2013). Maintaining empathy in medical school: It is possible. *Medical Teacher, 35*(12), 1002–1008.

Heyhoe, J., Birks, Y., Harrison, R., O'Hara, J. K., Cracknell, A., & Lawton, R. (2016). The role of emotion in patient safety: Are we brave enough to scratch beneath the surface? *Journal of the Royal Society of Medicine, 109*(2), 52–58.

Hilton, S., & Southgate, L. (2007). Professionalism in medical education. *Teaching and Teacher Education, 23*(3), 265–279.

Immordino-Yang, M. H., & Damasio, A. (2007). We feel, therefore we learn: The relevance of affective and social neuroscience to education. *Mind, Brain, and Education, 1*(1), 3–10.

Irving, P., & Dickson, D. (2004). Empathy: Towards a conceptual framework for health professionals. *International Journal of Health Care Quality Assurance, 17*(4), 212–220.

Isen, A. M., Rosenzweig, A. S., & Young, M. J. (1991). The influence of positive affect on clinical problem solving. *Medical Decision Making, 11*(3), 221–227.

Jennings, M. (2009). Medical student burnout: Interdisciplinary exploration and analysis. *Journal of Medical Humanities, 30*(4), 253–269.

Jones, A. M. (2010). Could kindness heal the NHS? *British Medical Journal, 340,* 1363.

Kearney, M. K., Weininger, R. B., Vachon, M. L., Harrison, R. L., & Mount, B. M. (2009). Self-care of physicians caring for patients at the end of life: "Being connected…a key to survival". *JAMA, 301*(11), 1155–1164.

Kerasidou, A., & Horn, R. (2016). Making space for empathy: Supporting doctors in the emotional labour of clinical care. *BMC Medical Ethics, 17*(1), 8–13.

Kim, S. S., Kaplowitz, S., & Johnston, M. V. (2004). The effects of physician empathy on patient satisfaction and compliance. *Evaluation and the Health Professions, 27*(3), 237–251.

Kozlowski, D., Hutchinson, M., Hurley, J., Rowley, J., & Sutherland, J. (2017). The role of emotion in clinical decision making: An integrative literature review. *BMC Medical Education, 17*(1), 255–268.

Krznaric, R. (2014). *Empathy: A Handbook for Revolution.* London: Random House.

Larson, E., & Yao, X. (2005). Clinical empathy as emotional labor in the patient-physician relationship. *JAMA, 293*(9), 1100–1106.
Levenson, R., Dewar, S., & Shepherd, S. (2008). *Understanding Doctors.* London: The Royal College of Physicians and The King's Fund.
Marshall, G. R. E., & Hooker, C. (2016). Empathy and affect: What can empathied bodies do? *Medical Humanities, 42,* 128–134.
Mayer, J. D., Salovey, P., & Caruso, D. R. (2008). Emotional intelligence: New ability or eclectic traits? *American Psychologist, 63*(6), 503–517.
McNaughton, N. (2013). Discourse(s) of emotion within medical education: The ever-present absence. *Medical Education, 47*(1), 71–79.
Meier, D. E., Back, A., & Morrison, R. (2001). The inner life of physicians and care of the seriously ill. *JAMA, 286*(23), 3007–3014.
Meitar, D., Karnieli-Miller, O., & Eidelman, S. (2009). The impact of senior medical students' personal difficulties on their communication patterns in breaking bad news. *Academic Medicine, 84*(11), 1582–1594.
Mercer, S. W., & Reynolds, W. J. (2002). Empathy and quality of care. *British Journal of General Practice, 52,* S9–S12.
Montgomery, K. (2006). *How Doctors Think: Clinical Judgment and the Practice of Medicine.* Oxford: Oxford University Press.
Osler, W. (1963). *Aequanimitas.* New York: Nortop.
Ratanawongsa, N., Teherani, A., & Hauer, K. E. (2005). Third-year medical students' experiences with dying patients during the internal medicine clerkship: A qualitative study of the informal curriculum. *Academic Medicine, 80*(7), 641–647.
Ricoeur, P. (1992). *Oneself as Another.* Chicago: University of Chicago Press.
Rogers, C. (1959). A theory of therapy, personality and interpersonal relationships as developed in the client-centered framework. In S. E. Koch (Ed.), *Psychology: A Study of Science—Formulations of the Person and the Social Context.* New York: McGraw-Hill.
Rogers, C. R. (1961). *On Becoming a Person.* London: Constable.
Rogers, W., & Ballantyne, A. (2010). Towards a practical definition of professional behaviour. *Journal of Medical Ethics, 36*(4), 250–254.
Salovey, P., Detweiler-Bedell, B., Detweiler-Bedell, J., & Mayer, J. (2008). Emotional intelligence. In M. Lewis, J. M. Haviland-Jones, & L. Feldman Barrett (Eds.), *Handbook of Emotions.* New York: Guilford Press.
Shapiro, J. (2008). Walking a mile in their patients' shoes: Empathy and othering in medical students' education. *Philosophy, Ethics, and Humanities in Medicine, 3*(1), 10–21.

Shapiro, J. (2011). Perspective: Does medical education promote professional alexithymia? A call for attending to the emotions of patients and self in medical training. *Academic Medicine, 86*(3), 326–332.
Shapiro, J. (2012). The paradox of teaching empathy in medical students. In J. Decety (Ed.), *Empathy: From Bench to Bedside.* Cambridge: MIT Press.
Shapiro, J. (2013). The feeling physician: Educating the emotions in medical training. *European Journal for Person Centered Healthcare, 1*(2), 310–316.
Spiro, H., Curnen, M., Peschel, E., & St. James, D. (1993). *Empathy and the Practice of Medicine.* New Haven: Yale University Press.
Tavakol, S., Dennick, R., & Tavakol, M. (2012). Medical students' understanding of empathy: A phenomenological study. *Medical Education, 46*(3) 306–316.
Warmington, S. (2012). Practising engagement: Infusing communication with empathy and compassion in medical students' clinical encounters. *Health, 16*(3), 327–342.
West, C. P., & Shanafelt, T. D. (2007). The influence of personal and environmental factors on professionalism in medical education. *BMC Medical Education, 7*(1), 29–38.
Winefield, H. R., & Chur-Hansen, A. (2000). Evaluating the outcome of communication skill teaching for entry-level medical students: Does knowledge of empathy increase? *Medical Education, 34*(2), 90–94.
Working Party of the Royal College of Physicians. (2005). Doctors in society: Medical professionalism in a changing world. *Clinical Medicine (London), 5,* S5–S40.
Zenasni, F., Boujut, E., Woerner, A., & Sultan, S. (2012). Burnout and empathy in primary care: Three hypotheses. *British Journal of General Practice, 62*(600), 346–347.

5
Enhancing Empathy

Overview

In this chapter, the students identified factors which encouraged empathy with patients. The main factor was their contact with patients, supported by an experienced clinician. They described aspects of teaching and support which they found encouraged empathy.

Patient Contact

Students asserted that face-to-face contact with patients was the most effective way of enhancing their empathy. They described experiences with patients in differing contexts; Gina found work experience in a deprived community instructive, as the doctors had radical approaches to social deprivation. Diana reflected that she did not meet socially deprived people in her life outside medicine, so felt less equipped to empathise with them. The students suggested that listening to patients' experiences and sharing their feelings enhanced their empathy.

D. I. Jeffrey, *Exploring Empathy with Medical Students*,
https://doi.org/10.1007/978-3-030-11211-0_5

> it was just completely different to anything I had seen in my placements here. [...]so that was very eye opening for me. (Gina, Year 6)

> I just don't meet people who are affected because their benefits are cut off. (Diana, Year 6)

> I think to enhance it [Empathy] on your way through medical school it is about taking on patient experiences and taking on what patients have told you about what they are feeling. (Kim, Year 4)

Despite her initial apprehension, Gina enjoyed the responsibility of conducting her own consultations in general practice. She came to appreciate that the patients did not expect her to know everything but valued her attention.

> It is still scary. But actually you realise more and more when you are interacting with people it is not that they expect you to know everything medically. They just a lot of time having someone there to listen and appreciate what is said. (Gina, Year 5)

Neville proposed that patient contact was central to developing empathy. He suggested that students should be like airline pilots, clocking in air miles, by logging their time spent with patients.

> I think medical students should have to do a certain number hours clocked off. (Neville, Year 5)

In the final years, students became focused on the needs of the patient rather than viewing them as learning resources. They described visiting the wards to listen to patients rather than 'hunting for signs.'

> I would love to hear from patients as actual people and not just feel like I am going to listen to the murmur and then [laugh] off to my next tutorial. (Gina, Year 6)

All the students expressed a wish for more time with patients, wanting to empathise with them and to learn more about their view of the world. Neville reflected on how patients had to repeat their story to different members of staff and students when they came to the hospital. He suggested that there might be a better way of understanding the patient's history than subjecting them to such repetition.

> They must have told that story to their GP, to the primary assessment doctor, to nurses who clerk them in, to the doctors that clerk them in, to the people on the ward, the consultant who sees them on the post take, it is seven or eight times they told story [...] must be so frustrated, [there] must be a better way [we]can do this. (Neville, Year 6)

In talking about their experiences with patients, students revealed their developing empathy. One clinical context which exemplified their empathy with patients was their first experience of a patient's death. Connie was unprepared for this but found that the experience made her reflect on her empathy as she tried to see things from the differing perspectives of the patient, family, doctors and nurses. She was impressed by the way the nurses' empathy extended to treating the patient's body with respect. She found the experience both shocking and moving. She was upset in recounting the circumstances of the patient's death that had occurred six months earlier. Connie described her feelings of sadness and shock of being in the patient's room immediately after he had died.

> to see this patient's slippers on the floor or clothes they laid out for the next day it is it is extremely apparent it like a juxtaposition like patient's expectation of life and the reality [of] their dead body lying there in the room that was very shocking [...] the patient's phone went off as they were trying to clean up the body. And it just this moment of silence in the room when everyone just pauses and kind of gasps as we hear the phone ringing knowing that this patient is never going to be able to pick that up. (Connie, Year 3)

It was clear from her story and others that although students were emotionally moved by a patient's death, these intimate experiences developed their empathy. They also talked about other patients whom they found both challenged, and yet paradoxically, enhanced their empathy. For example, Lisa and Amy said that they found it hard at times to empathise with psychiatric patients. While Paula claimed that she had become more empathetic as a result of her experience with patients with mental health problems.

> in terms of hallucinations or schizophrenia it is much more difficult to keep yourself in their shoes and appreciate what they are going through. (Lisa, Year 5)

> There were a lot of communication barriers and at first I felt really awkward. I was asking questions [...] and they would not be able to respond or understand and come to a point. (Amy, Year 5)

> it is easy initially to look at people who are suffering from depression and anxiety [...]and think that it self-inflicted. I have less of that opinion having seen it and I think actually that is an illness like any other illness. (Paula, Year 6)

Students described a range of emotional situations which challenged their empathy. They claimed that strong emotions made empathising more difficult, but found that after a pause for reflection, that they were able to explore the underlying reasons for the patient's distress. For example, Helen found it difficult to listen when a patient with advanced cancer was angry, but on reflection, she considered that the patient's anger was understandable.

> she was angry at the whole situation and just looking for things to blame. [...] she wasn't angry at the consultants really, she was just angry at the situation. I think it is understandable. (Helen, Year 1)

Cooper has commented how anger can impair one's receptivity to others (Cooper 2011).

Sometimes, students found it hard to empathise with patients whose illnesses had resulted from unhealthy lifestyles. Marilyn wondered why some obese patients did not care for themselves, but then she reflected on the possible underlying causes for their condition.

> my empathy completely disappeared for a few moments and I just thought, dear God you have gotten so fat you can't breathe. How does that happen? (Marilyn, Year 4)

> And then it took me second and I went, are they really unwell,? are they really depressed?, […] do they not have financial capacity? (Marilyn, Year 4)

Students also reflected on their feelings of helplessness, or even of guilt, when there was no obvious medical solution to the patient's problems.

> you want to be able to offer something [….] and when you can't that is quite a vulnerable place to be as well. You feel a bit guilty not being able to do something when you feel you should or could. (Paula, Year 6)

Sometimes it was the context of the clinical encounter which made empathising difficult but students found that addressing these situations enhanced their empathy. Ida described a consultation with a patient in handcuffs and was impressed that the doctor did not appear to be influenced by the man's crime.

> She [consultant] said she makes a point about not asking why they are accompanied by police because she doesn't want it to influence her care. (Ida, Year 4)

Students identified that their face-to-face contact with patients was one of the most influential ways of developing their empathy, which was also a prominent finding in other studies (Winseman et al. 2009; Egnew and Wilson 2010). In view of this finding, it is of particular concern that there appears to be a decline in bedside teaching (Elder and Verghese 2015). Medical students spend fewer hours in contact with patients, partly because of reduced inpatient stays, increasing class sizes and a greater use of simulated patients (Elder and Verghese 2015; Egnew and Wilson 2010).

In the early years, students enjoyed having time to spend with a limited number of patients (Ratanawongsa et al. 2005; Cutler et al. 2009). A systematic review concluded that early patient contact in undergraduate training enhanced empathy (Littlewood et al. 2005). Students in this study said that they had little patient contact in the first three years of their course which they described as being largely focused on the biomedical aspects of disease.

In their descriptions of contact with patients, students adopted a phenomenological stance. They wanted to connect with patients and talked about their interest in the patient's experience of their illness, confirming the findings of another qualitative study (Eikeland et al. 2014). Janssen et al. (2008) suggested that students should be supported, in their contact with patients, by experienced clinicians, with an opportunity for reflection and feedback. This was endorsed by Boudreau et al. (2007), who described an initiative in undergraduate education designed to put the patient and their illness at the heart of learning rather than focusing on the current disease-centred model of medical education. Another qualitative study of students' views concluded that students wanted opportunities to be directly observed by experienced clinicians in their relationships with patients and to be given feedback on their relationship skills (Egnew and Wilson 2010). Some students in my study reflected that it would be beneficial to have time with patients and to receive feedback, without feeling that they were being assessed by their clinical tutors. They described the pressure of assessment as fostering competition rather than empathy. Students stressed that contact with real patients rather than actors, or simulated patients, enhanced their empathy. Their views concurred with the findings in another study (Egnew and Wilson 2010).

Positive Role Models

The students found that positive role models enhanced their empathy. Diana described sitting in an outpatient clinic with a breast surgeon whom she considered to be an excellent role model. After breaking bad news of a diagnosis of breast cancer, he gave the patient time allowed her to go outside for a cigarette and ended the consultation with a hug. After the patient left, the surgeon took the time to explain to Diana why he had behaved in this way and this impressed her.

> he said afterwards when he sat down when she had left, he was in theory not supposed to hug patients but you could tell with that woman that was you needed to do as a human being. So I thought that was interesting that was the first time I had seen a surgeon talk about the importance of communication skills. (Diana, Year 4)

She also noted also that this surgeon extended his empathy to his colleagues by treating his team and juniors with respect.

> he was like that with his staff as well, the team was like that and trainees and everything. And so that was really inspirational for me. (Diana, Year 4)

Students identified a variety of characteristics of good role models, the most common of which were enthusiasm, humility and humanity.

> I think that is because they are sort of people that are passionate about the things. (Fiona, Year 2)

> it probably made her feel better because she [the consultant] kept on apologising probably feel guilty about not being able to do a perfect procedure. (Edward, Year 4)

Neville gave an example of a doctor who balanced connecting emotionally with a patient with her clinical decision making. Despite being upset, the doctor was empathetic as Neville described her sharing emotions with the patient and her family.

> I am sure that when she broke that news to the patient she was devastated at having to share the news with that patient. You could tell by the way she sat, her body language, her, her tone of voice, her choice of words and her clinical knowledge it was professional [...] at the same time I am here for you. I am not, not against you we are in this together. We are going work through it. (Neville, Year 4)

Kim suggested that good role models were the exceptions rather than the rule.

> you don't necessarily get as much exposure with to the ones who spend time with patients it depends on you stumbling on one of their clinics. (Kim, Year 6)

Paula, in a bedside teaching session, was impressed when the patient was included in the teaching by the consultant: this respected the patient's dignity and humanity. It also reflected the transition, in the students' eyes, of the patient as a resource for their learning to a unique human being.

> He also then said to the patient while we were there, "We are going to talk through your clinical history but I want you as a patient to listen and see if you pick up anything new from this". [...] I thought that was including a patient in that was a really nice way of making it a valuable time for them as well as us. (Paula, Year 5)

It seems that it is essential for students to have teachers who have reflected on empathy and appreciate the commitment required to become a good doctor (Schweller et al. 2017).

In the clinical years, students described their contact with positive role models as being inspirational and promoting their empathy which was also the finding of a survey of Canadian medical students (Byszewski et al. 2012). The students described how closely they watched clinical teachers in practice and how much this influenced their attitudes, which resonated with the findings of other studies (Haas and Shaffir 1987; Winseman et al. 2009; Curry et al. 2011).

However, one student in my study reported that such empathetic role models were the exception rather than the rule. A lack of positive role models has been suggested as a factor in causing students to have unrealistic expectations of how a doctor should behave (Chen et al. 2007). It has also been suggested that academic staff no longer build their reputations on clinical teaching expertise but are now judged on their ability to secure research grants and publish scientific papers (Elder and Verghese 2015). Authors have suggested that it was beneficial for clinical tutors to possess appropriate teaching skills and to improve their impact as positive role models (Burgess et al. 2015; Shapiro 2012).

The students described enthusiasm and empathy as characteristics of positive role models, which were attributes cited in another study (Burgess et al. 2015). They particularly appreciated when experienced doctors admitted their vulnerability and showed emotions. This was in contrast to the generally accepted notion that the expression of emotions by doctors was a sign of weakness or incompetence (Kerasidou and Horn 2016). Students claimed that when their teachers explicitly shared the emotional aspects of a situation it was a powerful way of learning (Passi et al. 2013). Rees et al. (2013) suggested that role models could use their stories to give examples of the dangers of suppressing emotion: burnout and detachment from the patient. Some of the role models the students described challenged stereotypes, such as a breast surgeon who demonstrated humanity, extending his respect for patients to the healthcare team.

Students described how positive role models also demonstrated ways of balancing connection and distancing with the patient to develop emotional regulation. Doctors who took time to attend to the students' welfare after a patient's death were also appreciated. These findings are similar to those in a study which found that students identified positive role models as doctors who encouraged them (Lempp and Seale 2004). Another study in the USA found excellent role models were those who stressed the importance of the doctor–patient relationship and taught psychosocial aspects of medicine (Wright et al. 1998). A qualitative study involved medical students asking patients 'What kind of doctor would you like me to be?' (Walsh et al. 2016). Patients overwhelmingly sought doctors with good personal qualities, including empathy and good communication skills, with only 8% of patients emphasising medical knowledge (Walsh et al. 2016).

Reflection

Students commented that the university encouraged reflection. For example, Olive said that she was encouraged to reflect on her experience but like several students found written reflection less helpful than discussing her experiences with others. Students talked about reflection in relation to empathy, feelings and stress. Bill said that there was an emphasis on a prescribed form of reflection which he did not find helpful in cultivating empathy.

> one of the problems with the university they always try to get you to reflect. (Bill, Year 3)

> they do teach you need to reflect you need to think more deeply about the kind of situations. (Olive, Year 1)

Connie enjoyed talking about her experiences, valuing verbal reflection and recognising a connection between reflection, self-awareness and empathy. She claimed that she had become more reflective as the course progressed. Sometimes she wrote a reflection as a way of coping with stress but preferred discussing it with other students. Fiona pointed out the advantages of reflecting on her experiences in enhancing learning. Neville described how reflection could be difficult but was necessary to enhance empathy.

> when I am feeling very overwhelmed I do write things down just keep an on and off diary when I am really struggling, but actually I don't know how much it helps. I would rather share it with someone because then I can get reassurance and I can get feedback. (Connie, Year 3)

> I think it is not just the exposure it is the reflecting on the exposure and what happened. (Fiona, Year 2)

> it is very hard to be reflective, it is very hard to look into oneself and criticise why and critically think […], why did I do that? and the more we talk about it I think the easier it becomes to analyse why and analyse empathy and the difficult things. (Neville, Year 4)

Neville reflected on this as he talked about seeing patients being given a diagnosis of lung cancer in the clinic. He reminded himself that every patient was unique and worthy of respect. He described part of empathising as pausing to reflect on the wider context of each patient

> as more and more people are given a diagnosis you do get that feeling that this is just another case but then you have go to stop yourself and

> say "No, no, this is a patient this is an individual with a family and much wider effects" and stopping and taking look at big picture is important. (Neville, Year 5)

A small number of students talked about how their own experience of illness had affected their empathy and their feelings about the course. For example, Marilyn talked about her mental health problems:

> But last semester I had an episode of depression which I needed medication for which took a long time to get and I think that it overshadowed being able to have a proper unbiased opinion of the course itself. (Marilyn, Year 1)

Fiona reflected that her own experience of illness had given her greater insight into the patient's perspective.

> I did have some health problems and it did make me realise how experiencing something yourself definitely changed the way […] you understood certain things more. I really don't want to go into it but I understood things more. (Fiona, Year 2)

The students described how their own experience of illness enhanced their empathy with patients and conversely how their lack of life experience limited it, findings which are supported in the literature (Woolf et al. 2007; DasGupta and Charon 2004). The students described how their empathy developed in challenging clinical situations such as in the care of dying patients and those with psychiatric disorders, which concurred with the findings of earlier qualitative studies (Ratanawongsa et al. 2005; Cutler et al. 2009).

The students claimed they had difficulties with written reflection but acknowledged that reflection was integral to the process of empathising. They said that they would value an opportunity to be able to talk to a patient, reflect and receive feedback without feeling that they were being assessed (Janssen et al. 2008). They valued the opportunity for verbal reflection, as an opportunity to share their concerns with colleagues and the teaching staff. Students described reflection as a strategy for coping with stress and so enhancing their empathy.

Providing students with a space for dialogue may be one way of nurturing reflection, empathy and of reducing stress (Ramesh 2013; Lutz et al. 2013; Branch 2010). Time for reflection is needed to help to make the implicit explicit (Cruess et al. 2008). Lutz et al. (2013), suggested that reflective practice required a secure space, a supportive group of students and an encouraging trainer. Other authors have suggested the need to develop a self-care plan to maintain empathy and prevent burnout. Such a plan might include mentoring, support, interests outside work, reflective writing and social networks (Sanchez-Reilly et al. 2013).

It appeared from the students' stories that empathy also had a spatial dimension, in terms of the closer the contact both physically and emotionally to the patient the deeper the empathy. From the students' stories, it seems that this close contact is balanced by the need to pause and step back to allow reflection on the patient's experience.

Students also talked about the teaching in the formal curriculum which they found had a positive influence on empathy.

Teaching

Despite the fact that students mostly claimed that there was little teaching on empathy in the curriculum, they discussed positive influences on their empathy of problem-based learning (PBL), communication skills training, simulation and lectures. Some students like Paula described a positive experience in an introductory lecture in which the lecturer referred to emotional problems.

> this semester introductory lecture was brilliantly done [...]he just spoke about it a little bit and mentioned occasions where he had been upset about a patient and had been told that was actually that made him a better doctor and he was encouraging us. (Paula, Year 5)

The students appreciated acknowledgement of emotions and receiving encouragement, but generally felt that formal communication skills training did not enhance their empathy. However, Ida claimed that working with simulated patients had helped her because she was able to get into role.

> I always find it quite easy to forget that it is just an actor and kind of properly get into and then it is really good fun. (Ida, Year 5)

Students identified the medical school's explicit commitment to empathy and altruism but paradoxically were exposed to an implicit culture of detachment and objectivity (Coulehan and Williams 2001). It seemed from their stories that the medical education process promoted emotional detachment, with little attention to the emotional needs of students (Jennings 2009; Shapiro 2012). Students also commented on the medical school culture which had both positive and negative influences on their empathy.

Medical School Culture

The culture, or ambience, of the medical school includes the organisational influences and the process of socialisation in becoming a doctor. The first-year students recalled how apprehensive they were before coming to university and how relieved they were to find a friendly atmosphere in the medical school. Most of the students commented on the friendliness of the other students throughout the course.

> university is about learning and becoming a doctor but my friends and I get on really well and that has been a big part of university as well. (Neville, Year 4)

In the clinical years, students compared the differing cultures of the larger, teaching hospitals with the smaller, more inclusive, peripheral units. Students claimed that sometimes they did not feel part of the team in the main teaching hospital but felt included in the smaller rural attachments.

> in the [large hospital] I just feel like a student. I am here to learn and I don't feel I am part of the team. (Amy, Year 5)

> Whereas in [the smaller hospital] he [the doctor] was very keen to involve me and introduced me as a doctor in training instead of medical student and he allowed me to help him. (Amy, Year 5)

Amy noticed that it was not just the students, but the patients, who were affected by the formality of the main teaching hospital and consequently were less likely to communicate.

> The patients [are] more chatty as well, talk to me and stuff. In [the large hospital] not so much. I think just difference in culture. (Amy, Year 5)

Kim was made more aware of the tensions which existed in the larger hospitals by observing that in smaller hospitals doctors and nurses had a better working relationship. Many students appreciated being valued by the hospital staff.

> the nurses were really friendly, the doctors were really friendly [...] it actually surprised me to find the nurse and doctor relationship was so good. (Kim, Year 6)

> I hadn't realised that there was such a tension in other places until I went there [smaller hospital] and all of a sudden everyone was on the same level and people were very much going out of their way to help others. (Kim, Year 6)

> they actually made me in some ways feel as part of their group because they will take me for a coffee when they had a break and things like that. (Jenny, Year 2)

The students described how their confidence improved when they felt part of a team. Kim remembered a nurse saying goodbye to her when she had finished her rural attachment on a Scottish island. Olive appreciated being valued by the medical school but was not sure whether an organisation could be described as empathetic.

> When I was leaving one the nurses said "you will always have a home here". It is things like that, the little things, that make a place really nice. (Kim Year 6)

> But from my understanding of empathy it's built around relationships and people. And so to say the medical school showing empathy, I can see individual professors and things if needed could show me empathy on

> an individual level for specific things [...] But I don't think students will look for that empathy from the medical school. (Olive, Year 2)

Students described how feeling valued, supported and part of a team enhanced their empathy. It seems that empathic treatment by others helps to develop empathy which in turn promotes moral decision-making (Cooper 2011). In discussing the ambience or culture of the medical school, students had little to say about positive influences on their empathy. They compared cultures in large teaching hospitals, which they perceived as formalised, and a more informal approach in smaller hospitals. In these smaller units, they found they were more likely to be valued and to be made to feel part of the team (Weaver et al. 2011). They suggested that such an environment increased their sense of well-being and their ability to empathise. The students' preference for smaller teaching hospitals was reflected in another study (Bennett et al. 2010). One student also noticed that the patients seemed more inclined to be open and comfortable in discussing their concerns in the smaller units.

Support

Lisa emphasised the importance of a supportive environment if she was to be empathetic to others. She pointed out that she was much better at empathising and exploring the patient's agenda when she felt comfortable. When she lacked confidence, she was more likely to stick solely to the medical agenda. Other students also linked improved self-confidence with enhanced empathy.

> I think that if you feel comfortable in what you are doing you can explore these ideas a lot more. Whereas if you are under confident, bit nervous then you much rather stick to then I am here to take your history and stick to that. (Lisa, Year 4)

> I think if you have got a good environment and feel supported you are more likely to have that interaction with patients. (Lisa, Year 4)

The variability of the support offered by the personal tutors in the medical school was a common theme.

> I think it depends who you have. [laughing] I definitely thinking about all supervisors I had before maybe two out of ten of them I would probably be happy to discuss something like that with. (Diana, Year 5)

> one of my flatmates had a member of family that died and it wasn't even slightly close member of family, it was the whole concept of him just dying just seemed to throw her and the university were absolutely brilliant. They just rearranged everything for her and sent her all the lectures. (Helen, Year 2)

Students described how they found dealing with dying patients a source of stress. Paula gave an example of a doctor providing informal support to a student after a patient's death, which she described as most helpful but unusual.

> She was quite taken aback that they said that because I have said that is rare. (Paula, Year 4)

However, it seemed that most of the students did not find their support in the personal tutor system but sought informal support from friends and family. Connie found that sharing experiences with other students was helpful because they seemed to care about her. Kim found support from being part of a clinical team and being able to share clinical problems.

Students also used other informal mechanisms of support such as reflection and trying to maintain a balance between their work and life outside medicine, a process described by Fiona as 'compartmentalisation'.

> I like to reflect on my feelings like write them down. I'm quite an expressive kind of personality so in the past when I had time, I would draw. (Amy, Year 4)

> Leave work at work and then that you have your home and your family and friend and people to support you and I think that is kind of compartments. (Fiona, Year 3)

A number of students derived their support from their religious faith.

> I have possibly quite a good set of support network at the local mosque. (Bill, Year 3)

> I am very involved in the church too and I think there is a lot of support there. (Paula, Year 4)

The university provided a personal tutor for each student but their experience with these tutors varied. Some described receiving good support but the students in this study found that they received little help from the tutor but instead approached family, friends or religious groups for informal support. They acknowledged that despite the university encouraging them to seek help, they were reluctant to access this for fears of being seen to be weak or that it might have an adverse consequence on their future careers (Jeffrey 2014).

Students valued being made to feel part of the clinical team and given responsibility. They found that when they were supported in such an environment they had the self-confidence to be more empathetic and to address emotional issues with the patient. Authors also suggest that increasing emotional support can reduce clinical detachment and foster true empathy (Austen 2016; Kerasidou and Horn 2016). Janssen et al. (2008) argued that to care for another, a person needed to receive care and support for themselves.

Key Points

- The students' views of the factors enhancing their empathy reflected the importance of the context of the clinical encounter in establishing empathy.
- Students claimed that contact with patients was the most effective way of developing their empathy.
- Positive role models inspired students to connect with patients.
- Students appreciated the opportunity for verbal reflection with their clinical teachers.
- Students stressed the value of support in enhancing their empathy.

References

Austen, L. (2016). Increasing emotional support for healthcare workers can rebalance clinical detachment and empathy. *British Journal of General Practice, 66,* 376–377.

Bennett, D., Kelly, M., & O'Flynn, S. (2010). Are the bigger hospitals better: DREEM on? *Irish Journal of Medical Science, 179,* 515–519.

Boudreau, J. D., Cassell, E., & Fuks, A. (2007). A healing curriculum. *Medical Education, 41,* 1193–1201.

Branch, W. T. (2010). The road to professionalism: Reflective practice and reflective learning. *Patient Education and Counseling, 80,* 327–332.

Burgess, A., Goulston, K., & Oates, K. (2015). Role modelling of clinical tutors: A focus group study among medical students. *BMC Medical Education, 15,* 17–26.

Byszewski, A., Hendelman, W., McGuinty, C., & Moineau, G. (2012). Wanted: Role models-medical students' perceptions of professionalism. *BMC Medical Education, 12,* 115–124.

Chen, D., Lew, R., Hershman, W., & Orlander, J. (2007). A cross-sectional measurement of medical student empathy. *Journal of General Internal Medicine, 22,* 1434–1438.

Cooper, B. (2011). *Empathy in Education: Engagement, Values and Achievement.* London: Bloomsbury Publishing.

Coulehan, J., & Williams, P. C. (2001). Vanquishing virtue: The impact of medical education. *Academic Medicine, 76,* 598–605.

Cruess, S. R., Cruess, R. L., & Steinert, Y. (2008). Role modelling—Making the most of a powerful teaching strategy. *BMJ, 336,* 718–721.

Curry, S. E., Cortland, C. I., & Graham, M. J. (2011). Role-modelling in the operating room: Medical student observations of exemplary behaviour. *Medical Education, 45,* 946–957.

Cutler, J., Harding, K., Mozian, S., Wright, L. L., Pica, A. G., Masters, S., et al. (2009). Discrediting the notion "working with 'crazies' will make you 'crazy'": Addressing stigma and enhancing empathy in medical student education. *Advances in Health Sciences Education, 14,* 487–502.

DasGupta, S., & Charon, R. (2004). Personal illness narratives: Using reflective writing to teach empathy. *Academic Medicine, 79,* 351–356.

Egnew, T. R., & Wilson, H. J. (2010). Faculty and medical students' perceptions of teaching and learning about the doctor–patient relationship. *Patient Education and Counseling, 79,* 199–206.

Eikeland, H. L., Ornes, K., Finset, A., & Pedersen, R. (2014). The physician's role and empathy—A qualitative study of third year medical students. *BMC Medical Education, 14,* 165–173.

Elder, A., & Verghese, A. (2015). Bedside matters—Putting the patient at the centre of teaching and learning. *The Journal of the Royal College of Physicians of Edinburgh, 45,* 186–187.

Haas, J., & Shaffir, W. (1987). *Becoming Doctors: The Adoption of a Cloak of Competence.* Greenwich, CT: JAI Press.

Janssen, A. L., Macleod, R. D., & Walker, S. T. (2008). Recognition, reflection, and role models: Critical elements in education about care in medicine. *Palliative & Supportive Care, 6,* 389–395.

Jeffrey, D. (2014). *Medical Mentoring: Supporting Students, Doctors in Training and General Practitioners.* London: Royal College of General Practitioners.

Jennings, M. (2009). Medical student burnout: Interdisciplinary exploration and analysis. *Journal of Medical Humanities, 30,* 253–269.

Kerasidou, A., & Horn, R. (2016). Making space for empathy: Supporting doctors in the emotional labour of clinical care. *BMC Medical Ethics, 17,* 8–13.

Lempp, H., & Seale, C. (2004). The hidden curriculum in undergraduate medical education: Qualitative study of medical students' perceptions of teaching. *BMJ, 329,* 770–773.

Littlewood, S., Ypinazar, V., Margolis, S. A., Scherpbier, A., Spencer, J., & Dornan, T. (2005). Early practical experience and the social responsiveness of clinical education: Systematic review. *BMJ, 331,* 387–391.

Lutz, G., Scheffer, C., Edelhaeuser, F., Tauschel, D., & Neumann, M. (2013). A reflective practice intervention for professional development, reduced stress and improved patient care—A qualitative developmental evaluation. *Patient Education and Counseling, 92,* 337–345.

Passi, V., Johnson, S., Peile, E., Wright, S., Hafferty, F., & Johnson, N. (2013). Doctor role modelling in medical education: BEME Guide No. 27. *Medical Teacher, 35,* e1422–e1436.

Ramesh, A. (2013). A call for reflection: Medical student driven effort to foster empathy and compassion. *Medical Teacher, 35,* 69–70.

Ratanawongsa, N., Teherani, A., & Hauer, K. E. (2005). Third-year medical students' experiences with dying patients during the internal medicine clerkship: A qualitative study of the informal curriculum. *Academic Medicine, 80,* 641–647.

Rees, C. E., Monrouxe, L. V., & McDonald, L. A. (2013). Narrative, emotion and action: Analysing 'most memorable' professionalism dilemmas. *Medical Education, 47,* 80–96.

Sanchez-Reilly, S., Morrison, L. J., Carey, E., Bernacki, R., O'Neill, L., Kapo, J., et al. (2013). Caring for oneself to care for others: Physicians and their self-care. *The Journal of Supportive Oncology*, 11, 75–81.
Schweller, M., Ribeiro, D. L., Celeri, E. V., & de Carvalho-Filho, M. A. (2017). Nurturing virtues of the medical profession: Does it enhance medical students' empathy? *International Journal of Medical Education*, 8, 262.
Shapiro, J. (2012). The paradox of teaching empathy in medical students. In J. Decety (Ed.), *Empathy: From Bench to Bedside.* Cambridge: MIT Press.
Walsh, S., Arnold, B., Pickwell-Smith, B., & Summers, B. (2016). What kind of doctor would you like me to be? *The Clinical Teacher,* 13, 98–101.
Weaver, R., Peters, K., Koch, J., & Wilson, I. (2011). 'Part of the team': Professional identity and social exclusivity in medical students. *Medical Education, 45,* 1220–1229.
Winseman, J., Malik, A., Morison, J., & Balkoski, V. (2009). Students' views on factors affecting empathy in medical education. *Academic Psychiatry, 33,* 484–491.
Woolf, K., Cave, J., McManus, I. C., & Dacre, J. E. (2007). It gives you an understanding you can't get from any book'. The relationship between medical students' and doctors' personal illness experiences and their performance: A qualitative and quantitative study. *BMC Medical Education, 7,* 50–58.
Wright, S. M., Kern, D. E., Kolodner, K., Howard, D. M., & Brancati, F. L. (1998). Attributes of excellent attending-physician role models. *New England Journal of Medicine, 339,* 1986–1993.

6
Barriers to Empathy: The Medical School Culture

Overview

This chapter addresses the hidden curriculum, the culture or ambience of the medical school. Many studies consider the medical school culture from the perspective of medical educators but few have investigated the views of students (Bandini et al. 2017). The context of the learning environment is critical for fostering a relational form of empathy. This exploration of the context or culture of the medical school revealed factors which the students described as inhibiting their empathy. The medical school studied is rated highly for research but receives low ratings from students for their teaching experience. In this chapter, many aspects of the hidden curriculum are made explicit. The links between student well-being, stress and empathy are discussed.

A Conforming Culture

Some students, in the early years, claimed that they were expected to follow a proscribed process in the medical school, which they described as a 'herd mentality'.

D. I. Jeffrey, *Exploring Empathy with Medical Students*,
https://doi.org/10.1007/978-3-030-11211-0_6

> It is almost herd mentality where you go along in your profession. (Bill, Year 3)

At the start of their course, they said that they lacked autonomy, but later maintained that they were left to fend for themselves. Marilyn, an overseas student, claimed that she had to conform to the mould of a British citizen, whom she described as being timid and formal. She claimed that the culture in the medical school discouraged interaction between students and teaching staff.

> I am stressed out by the lack of autonomy [...]I like to be in an environment where I felt people assume the best of me and I don't feel that. (Marilyn, Year 4)

> where for two years they [students] are spoon fed and then for the clinical years they are left to roam and, if you want help you have to go and ask for it. (Marilyn, Year 4)

> we want all of you to all act like in appropriate middle class British person and interact in that way which is hierarchy, confrontational avoidant. (Marilyn, Year 4)

As part of this conforming culture, students were inclined to keep silent for fear that their lack of medical knowledge would be exposed in their clinical teaching. Others expressed concerns that the conforming culture might inhibit some students from seeking support.

> it feels a little like a dystopian setting, you are in the medical school and they see all and they have a say in all and this is how you are to act XYZ.. I don't think it is healthy for all of us as students [...] .it discourages people who are struggling from seeking help or speaking out in a lot of aspects. (Gina, Year 6)

Students were reluctant to criticise or to seek support, findings shared in a study which identified the acceptance of hierarchy and the adoption of a ritualised professional identity as part of the hidden curriculum (Lempp and Seale 2004). It seemed that there was a disparity between the medical school's stated aspirations to promote diversity and the students' experiences of greater standardisation and conformity (Frost and Regehr 2013). It also appeared to the students that the faculty did not appear to acknowledge this tension and so it was not addressed (Frost and Regehr 2013).

A Lack of Empathy

If empathy is to be fostered, it might be expected that the medical school would be empathetic towards the students, but they told a different story. Bill claimed that the university was primarily interested in whether he passed exams rather than taking a personal interest in him. Fiona perceived empathy to be a 'buzz word' but questioned whether it was incorporated into the values of the medical school. Gina suggested that the medical school did not respect students as individuals.

> all the university, from my point of view, will see and know, Do I pass my exams? (Bill, Year 2)

> I think it is seen as a buzz word and potentially shown given quite high precedence, but whether that is translated into actual values I think is sometimes different. (Fiona, Year 3)

> That you have no chance to really feel like yourself. I struggle with feeling being a medic reconciles in medical school, the way we are examined, and the way we are, doesn't make allowances for you to be to be professional but in your own individual way that reflects you as a person. [....] it just feels very like a conveyor belt you got to stick to. (Gina, Year 6)

Other students also gave examples of their experiences of being treated without empathy by some medical school staff. Diana described the strain of looking after her terminally ill grandmother. She said that after her grandmother's death there was a lack of empathy from the staff of the teaching practice. She had to make up the time she had taken to attend the funeral.

> my grandmother died two weeks ago. And my placement was OK about it, but they were not great. [laughs] I said 'Sorry that I had to miss a day and half because I am going to funeral. [….] I will make up the time' and they said, 'OK, we will get rid of your day off then.' (Diana, Year 6)

Gina also described a harsh attitude to sickness absence by the medical school and suggested that this might be one reason why students avoided seeking support from the medical school.

> easy to see how people feel there is no hope so they wouldn't even bother trying approach medical school. (Gina, Year 6)

Ida resented deadlines and described being 'put through hoops' by the administration, which she found to be stressful.

> I do feel like they give us a lot of hoops to jump through. Things that are not necessary that for some reason that they want us to do. It does feel like they only do it to put some pressure on us. (Ida, Year 5)

A striking finding in this research was the students' widely held view that they were not shown empathy by the medical school. They described harsh attitudes of teaching staff to sickness absence and bereavement indicating that the medical school treated them, at times, with suspicion rather than as colleagues needing support (Back 2016, p. 32). Other authors have made the case for students needing more empathy from the faculty and their teachers before they can truly understand how to establish empathetic connections (Bayne 2011; Karnieli-Miller et al. 2011; Janssen and MacLeod 2010). A recent study showed how curricular change, in this case introduction of small group work and academic communities, enhanced the students' sense of connection with faculty (Brandl et al. 2017).

A Competitive Culture

Competition was described by students as the antithesis of collaboration and inhibited their empathy. They indicated that there was a competitive culture which was most noticeable in the early preclinical years but faded during the clinical years. They suggested that in the early years this reflected influences from school and the intense competition to enter medicine. Students noticed that the medical school encouraged competition from the outset.

> the body of medical students are competitive but I think that comes with getting into medicine is very competitive. (Edward, Year 2)

> The marks you get for first and second year they have a weighting towards the results when you graduate. (Bill, Year 3)

On the other hand, some students commented that there was also a sense of camaraderie as everyone was trying to get through the course. They were reassured by meeting older students who told them that they had struggled in the first year. Connie described the focus on exams as narcissistic rather than fostering empathy.

> I think trying so hard to do so well in exams can be incredibly narcissistic because it is focussing on your own performance so much. (Connie, Year 2)

Helen suggested that those students with the top grades were not necessarily the most empathetic.

> This sounds really bitchy but [they] do very well at medical school and you look at think I wouldn't want to talk to you, you are a bit scary. Yeah. But they get top grades. (Helen, Year 2)

Neville also implied that competition was not helpful in encouraging the development of empathetic doctors. Students felt pressure to perform well not just from the medical school, but from their families.

> Ultimately it does comes down to your grades and that sucks. That is really, really bad because not what it should be about in my opinion. We are in there to learn be good human beings. Learn to be good doctors to be able to look after patients yet we don't, [the] kind of environment some people create is unnecessary. (Neville, Year 4)

Students claimed that due to the lack of feedback from the medical school they resorted to comparing themselves with their peers, so further encouraging the competitive culture.

> if you had advice from higher up it would make it so much easier, because when you don't, the only reference points you have looking around at other people. (Helen, Year 3)

Gina suggested that highly competitive students risked burnout and gave an example of students trying to outdo their colleagues.

> I don't try and judge my achievements on how other people are doing. I try and step out of that and if you got into that it would be far too stressful environment and you would burn out [...] But there are certainly others who are like I want to be the best and would jump in front of you to get into a clinic or tell you it was elsewhere to get in. (Gina, Year 4)

> I know if they were struggling I guess they wouldn't necessarily let on because it can be quite a competitive dog- eat-dog attitude amongst medical students to each other sometimes. (Gina, Year 4)

However not everyone was competitive, Kim claimed that there was less competition in the clinical years. Paula was not so sure, concluding that there was great variability amongst the students.

> I think probably in first and second year it was because it was more lecture year, [...] I think being on clinical attachment you are not competitive. (Kim, Year 4)

> I think it hugely varies within our year probably. (Paula, Year 5)

There was a consensus that the competitive culture in the medical school was not conducive to developing empathy. Students felt that competition was encouraged by the medical school from the beginning of the course but tended to wane in the clinical years. They realised that their position in the year relative to their peers determined their chance of being appointed to one of the popular foundation year posts. Other studies have identified competition as a feature of the hidden curriculum (Lempp and Seale 2004; Nogueira-Martins et al. 2006). Marcum (2013) suggested that a competitive culture risked patient care. Authors have suggested that the level of empathy shown in competitive situations is manipulative and not of the deeper level of empathy required for moral development (Kozéki and Berghammer 1992). Moral empathy is of a higher order where concern for and understanding of the other is a long-term phenomenon (Cooper 2011).

Power

The students described power differentials which influenced their empathy in several contexts; the doctor–patient relationship, a fear of challenging authority, bullying and in the denigration of certain specialities. The hierarchy embedded in the medical school and in their clinical environment seemed to inhibit their empathy.

Fiona reflected that hierarchy did not always affect empathy adversely, since being regarded as having a lower status as a student could sometimes be an advantage. Some students argued that the relationship between empathy and power was complex and might depend more on the person's personality than their status.

> I think sometimes a patient might feel more comfortable and therefore more open and honest therefore empathy is kind of more facilitated with perhaps someone who is slightly more junior. (Fiona, Year 2)

Previous studies have shown that students perceived that they occupied a low position in the hierarchy of the medical school and experienced a pressure to compete (Lempp and Seale 2004; Ratanawongsa et al. 2005).

Many students claimed that they were unable to challenge some consultants who appeared to lack empathy for patients. Ida described feeling distressed when a patient's dignity was not respected by a consultant. She suggested that the students' reluctance to challenge their seniors was shared by some patients. Ida explained that she did not challenge the authority of consultants as she could not afford to jeopardise her progress and admitted that she was not aware of the whole picture. Students gave other examples where they felt distressed by a doctor's lack of empathy with a patient yet felt unable to say anything.

> It does vary some are more approachable than others. But for the most part it would be very difficult to question anything they did or say anything. (Paula, Year 4)

> he[consultant] wasn't the person you can tell that to but I have actually heard lots of other students tell very similar stories and I have not heard a single time they did actually say something to the doctor about it. I don't feel like as medical students we are in the right position to do. (Ida, Year 4)

> really uncomfortable.[…] And I was on the verge of wanting to say something to them as this is terrible. There were two others students there at the time and we both left, I don't know I just think that wasn't right that wasn't addressed. (Paula, Year 5)

The hierarchy within the medical school contributed to the conforming culture (Lempp and Seale 2004). Students described episodes when they were distressed to observe doctors behaving without empathy but felt constrained from challenging a consultant's behaviour (Rees and Monrouxe 2011). Students in other studies have described distress when they witnessed a lack of empathy and similarly felt powerless to challenge authority (Monrouxe et al. 2014; Rees et al. 2013; Monrouxe and Rees 2012).

Students referred to power differences when empathising with patients, reminiscent of Foucault's concept of 'the gaze' which described medical ways of knowing that put the student or doctor in the position of an observer of the patient and their disease (Bleakley and Bligh 2009). This positioning objectified the patient, making them a passive source of scientific interest and was dehumanising (Marshall and Hooker 2016). Some students described empathy as a bridge, between the doctor and patient, which tended to neutralise the power differences between them. However, if empathy is simply viewed as a desirable extra, and marginal to the more important biomedical aspects of disease, there is a risk of perpetuating the distanced medical 'gaze' (Marshall and Hooker 2016). There was also a risk that empathy could become a tool by which the doctor exercised power (Mayes 2009). For instance, one student described how she used empathy as a tool to effect changes in a patient's smoking habit.

The students were made aware of a hierarchy of specialities by some teachers. For example, Gina described derogatory comments about general practice, illustrating the low esteem for this speciality which was perpetuated in the medical culture and absorbed by some students.

> There is still that attitude that it is not academic to be a GP, it is an easy option. People only do it for work life balance. Women go and do it so they can have babies and work part time that kind attitude that kind of dismissive overgeneralised thought. And you do see it in your peers and you do see it in teaching. (Gina, Year 6)

Baker et al. (2016) speculated that the widespread denigration of general practice in medical schools might contribute to the problem of recruitment to the speciality. The medical school in this study had a low rate of graduates entering general practice perhaps reflecting its reputation for biomedical scientific research (Goldacre et al. 2004). It is paradoxical that specialities with low levels of patient contact tend to be regarded as the most prestigious (Hinze 1999). High prestige specialties such as surgery have been found to attract less empathetic doctors and low prestige specialties, such as general practice or palliative care, more empathetic doctors (Hojat et al. 2005).

Power can be abused and some students described being bullied or humiliated. Lisa gave an example, when she had been humiliated on a ward round by a cardiologist and felt she could not return to the patient. Lisa was still visibly distressed as she recounted this experience. She reflected that her humiliation had made her resolved not to behave in this way in the future with her colleagues.

> But she introduced me and saying that I was going to be a doctor in a couple years' time and it was rather scary since I got to this stage and couldn't read an ECG and that kind of thing. So it makes you feel a bit small [nervous laugh]. (Lisa, Year 4)

> it is not very nice, no. It kind played on my mind the rest of the day. And obviously two days later it is still [...] I did find as well that I don't feel like I could then go back to that patient and have a normal conversation. (Lisa Year 4)

Paula described consultants who were intimidating and embarrassed staff and students. She maintained that this humiliation was not malicious. On the other hand, Marilyn claimed that she was not afraid to speak out but was aware that this did not fit in with the university's wish to retain a hierarchy in the medical school.

> there are intimidating consultants and I have seen them embarrass junior doctors for example sometimes medical students, but never in a malicious way. (Paula, Year 4)

> I am outspoken, [...] and people don't like that. People don't like it when you look at them like you are on same level. Like you are just two people. They want a hierarchy. (Marilyn, Year 4)

Abuse of power by humiliation or bullying had the effect of undermining the students' confidence and empathy with patients (Lempp and Seale 2004). A study of medical students in the UK revealed that 20% of students experienced bullying on their clinical attachment (Timm 2014). Rees and Monrouxe (2011) found that commonly students took no action in response to bullying. It seems to some authors and to the students that awareness by the medical faculty of abuse of students in medical education had resulted in little effective change (Rees and Monrouxe 2011; Timm 2014).

Just as students described feeling intimidated by consultants and failing to raise their concerns, some patients were intimidated by doctors. Kim implied that both the consultants and students are on a spectrum of approachability.

> I think there is probably spectrum of approachability. (Kim, Year 5)

This view is supported by research linking being open to experiences, having an agreeable personality and empathy (Costa et al. 2014).

Time: Balancing Empathy and Efficiency

Many students suggested that establishing empathy required spending an appropriate amount of time with the patient.

> I think when you have more time with your patients you can empathise with them more because you learn more about them. And you learn more about them as people. (Kim, Year 6)

In the clinical years, the students claimed that in order to practise efficiently, they had to spend less time with patients. It was apparent that a tension existed between empathy and efficiency. They also claimed that a shortage of time created stress, which reduced their empathy. Bill described how a lack of time made him adopt a more detached manner, becoming focused on his own behaviour rather than on the patient.

> when I was under time constraint and when I was thinking over things in my head it was almost less about me examining the patient but more me running over my head, Have I done this correctly ? (Bill, Year 3)

Kim argued that exploring the patient's feelings would take more time. She found it unsatisfactory when she neglected to explore the patient's emotional needs, claiming that she would feel inhibited if allowed only ten minutes for a consultation. She wondered whether people who did not explore feelings did not necessarily lack time but lacked an empathetic approach.

> I don't think I would appreciate it as much if it was just ten minutes per clinic appointment. But then maybe the people that don't explore those type of things don't find it stressful to not explore that. I suppose that whether what causes them not to go into it in the first place whether it is time constraint or whether an innate issue. (Kim, Year 4)

Some students in the clinical years described a culture of a lack of time; Gina noticed that the workload seemed to squeeze out the human aspects of care during her general practice experience.

> just seeing that in action and just how relentless it is. It feels very like something is lost and then the opportunities you do have where you know that bit of extra time and a human touch would be beneficial to that person is often not possible, which is really sad. (Gina, Year 6)

Several students were distressed by rapid ward rounds in surgical specialities. For instance, Lisa was aware that psychological issues were not addressed in any depth on some surgical ward rounds. Neville noticed the speed of some orthopaedic surgeons' ward rounds left some elderly patients confused. He suggested that it was shortage of time which constrained doctors from giving a satisfactory level of psychosocial care.

> they are going through their ward round they are desperate to get to theatre. [....] I think it is mostly time or people just, for them going back to surgery, what is important is to fix this broken leg, not worry they are not you know feeling a bit down on the side anything like that. (Lisa, Year 5)

> the lack of communication, the brashness, or the speediness of their ward round leaves patients confused. They talk amongst themselves rather than address the patient and I thought that was quite poor. [.....] I just wish they had given her more time and actually talked to her rather to themselves. (Neville, Year 6)

> I think all the doctors I have seen are very caring individuals and they want to care but they don't have the time to do that. [...] I genuinely do feel unfortunately that we don't give patients that aspect of the care. [...] But us as doctors are notoriously bad at not giving patients enough time. (Neville, Year 6)

In bedside teaching, the emphasis was also on efficiency rather than empathy. Kim explained how her feedback to a consultant about a patient's history had to be concise and focus on the medical issues. She suggested that spending time with a patient was not valued by the tutors.

> there is very much a time restriction there and you do have to learn to be very concise especially you are being taught how to feed back to a consultant. (Kim, Year 5)

> I don't think it is really said you go and spend any time with patient it is a very valuable thing to do. (Kim, Year 5)

Students were concerned that the drive for efficiency not only threatened their empathy but could lead to clinical errors.

> You have to be efficient with the way manage your time and therefore empathy gets thrown to the back. (Amy, Year 6)
>
> Whereas the time pressured and you miss things. (Kim, Year 6)
>
> time and maybe having other things on your mind not concentrating as fully as you should and picking up on cues. (Lisa, Year 6)

Time shortage was also related to stress and to reducing empathy. Students highlighted how time and stress affected their empathy.

> When you have less time you don't get to know people and you get stressed. (Kim, Year 6)

Most of the students in the clinical years felt that their empathy was inhibited by a lack of time. It could be questioned whether it is reasonable to expect empathetic relationships with patients given the demands of medical practice in the NHS today (Halpern 2014). Students reflected on their experiences in the early years when they met very few patients but had plenty of time to listen to them and contrasted this with the clinical years when they perceived a tension between empathy and efficiency. Other qualitative studies on medical students' empathy have also identified a shortage of time as a barrier to empathy (Ratanawongsa et al. 2005; Nogueira-Martins et al. 2006; Tavakol et al. 2012; Eikeland et al. 2014). Conversely, students claimed that having more time helped to establish their connection with patients (Cutler et al. 2009).

Students described a link between their perceived lack of time and stress which in turn reduced their empathy. They gave descriptions of patients being treated abruptly on ward rounds and described how distressing they found this. There was uncertainty about the extent to which distancing behaviour was due to a shortage of time or to the doctor's personality.

Students reported how they felt rushed when presenting a patient's story on a ward round, where the emphasis was on stating medical facts concisely and so neglected psychosocial issues. They observed that a shortage of time could lead to medical errors. Verghese (2008) has argued that spending time with patients, listening and carefully examining them might avoid unnecessary tests and procedures. Bauer (2008) suggested that while fast medicine is appropriate in emergency situations, there may be a place for slow medicine in many of the illnesses which evolve chronically. Wear et al. (2014) also challenged the culture of speed in medical education and practice. They described a 'slow medical education' where instead of a rush to efficiency, there was a commitment by the faculty to provide time for students to reflect about their experiences (Wear et al. 2014).

Christakis and Feudtner (1997) proposed that a possible factor in the dehumanising of doctors and students was the transient nature of relationships during training. They argued that temporary relationships lacked human connection both with patients and colleagues resulting in a pressure to do something. In this way, 'efficient' doctors may become alienated from patients (Christakis and Feudtner 1997). Furthermore, they indicated that students who do spend time with patients risk being regarded as inefficient (Christakis and Feudtner 1997). It has been argued that a doctor should spend more time in establishing empathetic relationships and that those responsible for the doctor's workload should restructure their timetables to allow for such empathy (Hardy 2017).

The students' conversations around levels of empathy suggested a way forward in this dilemma (Cooper 2011). Sometimes understanding a patient's situation appropriately to meet their needs did not require the clinician to engage in a deeper level of empathy than simply acknowledging the patient as a human being who is valued (Halpern 2014). A relational view of empathy acknowledges that appropriate empathy can be achieved by different levels of empathising depending on the clinical situation.

Finally, it can be argued that allowing the patient to create a narrative is not as time-consuming as may be assumed (Hardy 2017). It has been shown that allowing a patient to establish their story takes approximately two minutes, for 78% of those patients (Langewitz et al. 2002). However, Marvel et al. (1999) showed that doctors interrupted the patient's story after a mean of 23 seconds. There is, therefore, scope for doctors who possess 'narrative competence' to allow patients to complete their story in a short time within an empathetic relationship.

The context of their clinical work also affected their ability to be empathetic, particularly when they were busy or lacked privacy (Tavakol et al. 2012). Lack of time was commonly cited as a challenge for establishing empathy with patients (Ratanawongsa et al. 2005; Tavakol et al. 2012; Eikeland et al. 2014).

Allen et al. (2008) undertook a qualitative study exploring the culture of the medical school and recruited 19 second-year medical students to keep weekly journal entries during the first five months of their medical apprenticeship. The themes that emerged from their reflections included a competing discourse between empathy and efficiency, the objectification of patients, the power of the medical hierarchy and the institutionalised practice of 'wounding' (Allen et al. 2008). The latter referred to routine practices where the patient was subjected to indignity or harm in the process of the students' learning (Allen et al. 2008).

Stress

The students agreed that they were less empathetic when they felt stressed. They described some effects of stress, causing them to withdraw from patients and to lose concentration.

> I can feel less willing to listen to long winded anecdotes. (Ida, Year 6)

> you can't actually concentrate on the patient. (Olive, Year 1)

The majority of students saw stress as unhelpful, but a few reflected that in some situations being stressed might create a bond with the patient.

> You see other people who are going through difficulties and because you know that you are suffering or having a hard time yourself you feel much more connected to that person. (Connie, Year 2)

Students identified many causes of stress including shortage of time, workload, assessment and competition. They also identified clinical issues which caused them stress, such as caring for dying patients, observing poor practice and their own mental health problems. Lisa described a cycle in which a doctor with less time became stressed had less empathy and spent less time with the patient. She suggested that a combination of the workload, time pressures and stress encouraged doctors to behave without empathy. Most students talked about the stress of exams and assessment.

> just the work load, the situation, the amount of stress on you and how much you have got to get through that dictate how long you can spend. (Lisa, Year 4)

> Last semester at exam time I think I must have been incredible stressed yeah. [...]got very little sleep and saw very little of the outside world, of the outdoors in general. That was very much an environment cultivated by all the medical students. (Olive, Year 2)

Amy talked of her stress when a patient she knew died unexpectedly. She felt sad and guilty and found it difficult to find anyone with whom to share her feelings.

> I went on Sunday to check how he did and unfortunately they told me he passed away the night before and I just felt really sad. (Amy, Year 5)

> I still remember what I said to the patient the day before surgery. I told him don't worry you will be fine. You will be in good hands and I reflect on what I said. Hmm. (Amy, Year 5)

Diana claimed that the medical culture demanded that they concealed their stress from others, sometimes even physically, hiding in a 'crying cupboard'.

> these other students or junior doctors had very much required a 'crying cupboard' and found one and it had become a thing in the department that existed. (Diana, Year 6)

A number of students talked about their own mental health during the course including depression, grieving, anxiety and disillusionment.

> I have been either depressed or physically a bit unwell or incredibly stressed or any combination thereof plus sleep deprivation. (Marilyn, Year 4)

> I was struggling towards the end of second year when I realised that like it is all about management, management treatment, management, blah, investigation so it was very core science. (Amy, Year 4)

> It was all over the place. Doing a placement on top of that wasn't that great obviously just because it was a tough few weeks. (Diana, Year 6)

The students claimed that they tended to distance themselves from patients when they felt stressed. The heavy clinical workload and shortage of time led to reduced empathy and a risk of clinical errors and further stress, findings that were confirmed in a survey of practising physicians (Ahrweiler et al. 2014).

Although some stress is a normal part of training, it can be associated with both psychological and physical illness (Dyrbye et al. 2005, 2010). The authors suggested that strategies for coping with stress that involved detachment from the patients correlated with depression and anxiety and poor mental health. In contrast, strategies that involved engagement, support and expression of emotion enabled students to respond in a healthy way (Dyrbye et al. 2005). This way of addressing stress was described by Antonovsky as a salutogenic approach to well-being (Antonovsky 1996). The students described a culture which discouraged any admission of stress. One student talked about a cupboard on a ward which was known by the doctors and students as the 'crying cupboard', inferring it was necessary to hide away on one's own rather than to display emotion or to seek support.

Students were concerned that by connecting emotionally with some patients that they might be at risk of burnout. Burnout, a stress-related syndrome, is characterised by exhaustion, depersonalisation and a diminished sense of accomplishment and was related to lower medical student empathy (Brazeau et al. 2010; Thomas et al. 2007). On the other hand, there was evidence that well-being was positively correlated with higher levels of empathy (Thomas et al. 2007). Recent research suggests that high levels of empathic concern are associated with low levels of burnout. Conversely, high levels of personal distress are linked to high levels of burnout (von Harscher et al. 2018). Jennings (2009), maintained that burnout arose when the medical culture was unresponsive to people, which concurred with the students' perceptions of not being shown empathy by the medical school.

Zenasni et al. (2012) suggested three alternative hypotheses in exploring the possible relationships between empathy and burnout; burnout prevents empathy, empathy creates burnout and empathy prevents burnout. There are quantitative studies which show that burnout is associated with a decline in empathy (Shanafelt et al. 2005; Brazeau et al. 2010; Paro et al. 2014). There is a belief that empathy can lead to burnout which is one reason for the prevalent medical culture of detached concern (Zenasni et al. 2012; Halpern 2001). However, adopting 'detached concern' rather than protecting the student from stress may instead lead to burnout (Ekman and Halpern 2015). The literature suggests that empathy prevents burnout since it is claimed that emotionally engaged physicians were fulfilled and so had greater effectiveness (Halpern 2001). One study found that oncologists who incorporated both biomedical and psychological approaches viewed provision of end-of-life care as satisfying (Jackson et al. 2008). In contrast, participants who described primarily a biomedical role reported a more distant relationship with the patient and a sense of failure (Jackson et al. 2008). The authors concluded that the latter group had an increased risk of burnout, while those who connected empathetically were protected from burnout (Jackson et al. 2008). Other research also supported this view (Harrison and Westwood 2009; Kearney et al. 2009).

It appeared from these studies that burnout resulted in a decline in empathy and that empathy may protect against distress and burnout. However, some students were concerned that by sharing feelings and connecting emotionally with patients that they risked burnout, reflecting a prevalent belief in medical practice (Zenasni et al. 2012; Halpern 2001). However, at the same time most said that they would not feel fulfilled if they had to work in a detached manner a view, reflected in Epstein's study (Epstein 2014).

The students described resilience as facilitating their engagement with patients although some were concerned it implied some distancing. Resilience can be seen as more than the ability to adapt to change and achieve goals in the face of adversity (Epstein 2014). Resilience can also involve empathy, humility and managing uncertainty (Epstein 2014).

The need for personal distance from patients with the aim of self-protection can lead to attitudes of cynicism and loss of empathy (Schweller et al. 2017). Previous research has shown that students responded to stress by distancing themselves from patients to avoid being overwhelmed by emotions (Cutler et al. 2009; Eikeland et al. 2014). Some students described becoming accustomed to distress and even developing indifference (Eikeland et al. 2014). Cynicism was perceived by some students as an acceptable means of dealing with stress, rather than a cause for concern (Eikeland et al. 2014).

Authors have argued that if students and doctors are to provide empathetic care they should optimally be in a positive frame of mind and not stressed (Shanafelt et al. 2005; Zenasni et al. 2012). However, distress is commonly reported in medical students (Firth-Cozens 2001). Stress may also have a negative influence on empathy if students use coping strategies such as distancing (Dyrbye et al. 2005; Neumann et al. 2011).

Student distress has been linked to factors in the hidden curriculum; abuse by superiors, vulnerability, lack of support, and high workload (Lempp and Seale 2004). Neumann et al. (2011) speculated about factors in the formal curriculum contributing to distress inappropriate learning environments, negative role models and lack of continuity (Neumann et al. 2011).

Lack of Support

Students indicated that stress influenced their empathy; therefore, it was relevant to listen to their views of the support offered by the medical school. They described the support as variable, depending on the individual personal tutor. Edward spoke for several students who had not found their personal tutor helpful.

> Some people say the exactly same thing as me, it is less than useless. Some people say they are fantastic. (Edward, Year 2)

Several students had not even met their personal tutor and some had experienced unhelpful meetings. For example, Helen described a meeting with a personal tutor who was pleasant, but so distracted by work that she felt guilty for bothering him.

> I have not seen mine yet. I think no one I have spoken to have ever said they would go to their personal tutor. (Olive, Year 2)

> I felt bad for him because he is an acute medicine consultant [...] He seemed really busy and he welcomed me into his office and there are stacks of paper everywhere and his pager kept going off and then but he was really nice tried to ignore it and stuff and asking how are you feeling. Clearly like just go back on the ward [laughing]. (Helen, Year 1)

Amy did not receive any support after a patient died unexpectedly.

> I did go back to ask the surgeon what when wrong and was it expected? He just gave a sigh and 'that is what happens'. And I was like oh, OK. He does not want to talk more about it. (Amy, Year 5)

Students said that they were reluctant to seek support from personal tutors but preferred informal sources of support. Connie said that she did not want to burden someone else with her problems. Whereas in first year she might have gone to someone and to vent her feelings, she was now conscious of their needs and was more resilient.

> I think part of it is also needing to learn to not burden people too much with your own emotions, because it can be burden. (Connie, Year 3)

Although personal tutors were available to provide support, students felt there was a stigma in seeking support and some students were worried that it might impact adversely on their future careers.

> I think you've probably got a cohort of people who don't probably like to admit they are struggling. (Fiona, Year 3)

> I think people worry about seeking support is how it may impact future careers. (Gina, Year 4)

In contrast, others accepted that seeking support was sensible and suggested that the university needed to emphasise the confidentiality of the support system.

> being able to seek support shows a level of maturity of mind, it is a good thing that people actually address things rather get to the point they are putting themselves or others, in a risky situation. (Gina, Year 4)

Students also identified administrative barriers in arranging a meeting with their tutors and a lack of clarity about the provision of pastoral support. The students claimed that there was a lack of guidance from the university on coping with emotional stress and they would welcome more support.

> I don't know if most people are comfortable putting it in the words in an email that they need help. I think it formalises something they don't want to be formal. (Bill, Year 3)

> the personal tutor first of all says, "I am not your mum. So if you have got worries, I am not the one who has to deal with this. (Olive, Year 3)

> I don't think anything is said, medicine is really tough sometimes and this is how you do it and this is the support network that is here. [...] Even if it is, 'Here is method how to switch off at the end of the day take five minutes.' (Kim, Year 5)

Since students identified stress as a prominent inhibitor of empathy, the provision of support for students would appear to be essential. Providing support for medical students is a GMC requirement of a medical school (General Medical Council 2009). Jennings (2009) claimed that student burnout can be attributed to a medical school culture that failed to value medical students. He called for medical schools to create learning environments that respected the integrity of students and nurtured them as professionals and people (Jennings 2009). This suggestion was supported by Benbassat (2014), who concluded, in a narrative review of the literature on well-being, that medical training caused emotional distress. Other authors have also made the case for a nurturing learning environment in medical schools (Dyrbye et al. 2005).

Students agreed that the level of support provided by the medical school depended largely on the personality of the individual personal tutor. They noted that some tutors were uncertain of their role. The students acknowledged that the university provided support but they expressed concerns about appearing weak or that seeking support might affect their career progression. Others were concerned about the confidentiality of the support system and found administrative barriers in arranging meetings with busy clinicians. Other authors also found that support offered by the medical school may not be accessed by students for fear of stigma or the effect on their grades (Chew-Graham et al. 2003). Students in another study appreciated the opportunity to discuss difficult issues in relating to patients in an informal setting but students in my research reported difficulty in accessing such support (Nogueira-Martins et al. 2006).

Social support is essential for maintaining physical and mental health with the lack of support being a risk factor for psychological illness (Cacioppo et al. 2011; Reblin and Uchino 2008; Ozbay et al. 2007). There was little in the literature that described empathy between the faculty and medical students (Kerasidou and Horn 2016). Students need to develop effective mechanisms of self-care and healthy ways of relieving stress to maintain their well-being (Coulehan and Williams 2003; Kerasidou and Horn 2016).

Other Influences in the Medical School Culture

The students spoke about other factors contributing to the medical school culture including alcohol, loneliness and social media.

A culture of alcohol consumption by some medical students affected their socialisation, particularly in the first two years of the course.

Marilyn suggested the drinking culture did not exclude students from socialising, but Connie felt excluded by it.

> I don't want to bring it up, but these students drink so much.[laughing] I mean I can't imagine it to be professional to drink on a Wednesday night and go out and then get a lecture the next morning. But they do. (Marilyn, Year 2)

> I think a lot events centre around alcohol but I think the students are a very friendly bunch. So if someone came along and wanted to have a good time and just wasn't drinking they wouldn't be pushed into it. (Marilyn, Year 2)

> I definitely feel like there are a lot of activities I can't partake in because of the amount of drinking. (Connie, Year 1)

Diana gave a vivid example of facilitating a tutorial with six students who were still under the influence of alcohol.

> I am a PBL tutor [...] I come to a tutorial next morning and I am trying to work and all of my six students are hungover or still drunk. (Diana, Year 5)

One of the surprising findings in this study was that some students reported loneliness to be a significant problem despite describing their peer group as friendly. Some overseas students in particular found it difficult to integrate with their peers, describing how cliques were established in the medical school.

> after the introduction week, almost everyone seemed to have their own little group. (Jenny, Year 1)

> And at first I guess coming from international background you want to come and mingle with everyone and that was a big struggle because I don't do alcohol, I don't go clubs, I don't pub whatever, and as hard, I guess as hard as you try to fit in, it is difficult when [...] there is nothing I can talk about. (Amy, Year 4)

Students were dismissive of the influence of social media on their ability to empathise. They used social media to arrange meetings and share work information. They claimed that social media presented an unreal image of people and suggested that it was unwise to share emotional information. They implied that social media did not enhance their empathy. However, since it provided anonymity, Marilyn suggested it might enable people to share concerns, but she described an episode of bullying on Facebook.

> I think it makes easier for practical people to communicate […] but I don't think it makes you more connected. (Edward, Year 2)

> it is very different to face to face communication. […] people don't put their life and soul and personal emotions on social media which I think is a very good thing. (Fiona, Year 2)

> you paint a picture of yourself on social media that is not the same as who you are. (Paula, Year 5)

> It lends itself to people opening up to other people when they might be too nervous. It lends itself to people to be mean to each other. It lends people to asking for help when they might not otherwise do. So it is not a simple good or bad. (Marilyn, Year 2)

> last week one of the students got really drunk and decided it would be funny to post an incredibly, incredibly rude comment on Facebook on the medics page (Marilyn, Year 1)

It was surprising that some students talked about a drinking culture in the early years which alienated them from social events. A study of second-year students at one medical school found that 50% of medical students reported exceeding recommended safe levels of alcohol consumption (Pickard et al. 2000). International students in particular felt socially isolated partly because they did not drink alcohol. Three students in the study admitted that they felt lonely, even in the final years of the course.

Students were ambivalent about the use of social media, being wary of any emotional self-disclosure, and one student described being bullied on social media. Students claimed that they used social media to share teaching resources and arrange meetings. There have been concerns that young people are becoming less empathetic as a result of using social media (Twenge 2013; Konrath et al. 2010). However, a survey of Dutch adolescents suggested that using social media improved both their cognitive and affective empathy (Vossen and Valkenburg 2016). A survey of medical students at one university found that social media use was widespread but the majority were unaware of GMC guidance on its appropriate use (Kang et al. 2015; General Medical Council 2013).

Key Points

- The students identified key areas in the medical school culture which they described as barriers to their empathy: a conforming culture, a lack of empathy for students, a shortage of time and a culture of alcohol which have not been widely reported in the medical education literature in relation to empathy.
- The study confirmed earlier reports of the influence of competition, hierarchy, stress and the need for support.
- Awareness of these influences does not appear to have led to many changes in the medical school culture (Rees and Monrouxe 2011).

References

Ahrweiler, F., Neumann, M., Goldblatt, H., Hahn, E. G., & Scheffer, C. (2014). Determinants of physician empathy during medical education: Hypothetical conclusions from an exploratory qualitative survey of practicing physicians. *BMC Medical Education, 14,* 122–134.

Allen, D., Wainwright, M., Mount, B., & Hutchinson, T. (2008). The wounding path to becoming healers: Medical students' apprenticeship experiences. *Medical Teacher, 30,* 260–264.

Antonovsky, A. (1996). The salutogenic model as a theory to guide health promotion. *Health Promotion International, 11,* 11–18.

Back, L. (2016). *Academic Diary: Or Why Higher Education Still Matters*. London: Goldsmiths.
Baker, M., Wessely, S., & Openshaw, D. (2016). Not such friendly banter? GPs and psychiatrists against the systematic denigration of their specialties. *British Journal of General Practise, 66*, 508–509.
Bandini, J., Mitchell, C., Epstein-Peterson, Z. D., Amobi, A., Cahill, J., Peteet, J., et al. (2017). Student and faculty reflections of the hidden curriculum: How does the hidden curriculum shape students' medical training and professionalization? *American Journal of Hospice and Palliative Medicine, 34*, 57–63.
Bauer, J. L. (2008). Slow medicine. *The Journal of Alternative and Complementary Medicine, 14*, 891–892.
Bayne, H. B. (2011). Training medical students in empathic communication. *The Journal for Specialists in Group Work, 36*, 316–329.
Benbassat, J. (2014). Changes in wellbeing and professional values among medical undergraduate students: A narrative review of the literature. *Advances in Health Sciences Education, 19*, 597–610.
Bleakley, A., & Bligh, J. (2009). Who can resist Foucault? *Journal of Medicine and Philosophy, 34*, 368–383.
Brandl, K., Schneid, S. D., Smith, S., Winegarden, B., Mandel, J., & Kelly, C. J. (2017). Small group activities within academic communities improve the connectedness of students and faculty. *Medical Teacher, 39*(8), 1–7.
Brazeau, C., Schroeder, R., Rovi, S., & Boyd, L. (2010). Relationships between medical student burnout, empathy, and professionalism climate. *Academic Medicine, 85*, 33–36.
Cacioppo, J. T., Hawkley, L. C., Norman, G. J., & Berntson, G. G. (2011). Social isolation. *Annals of the New York Academy of Sciences, 1231*, 17–22.
Chew-Graham, C. A., Rogers, A., & Yassin, N. (2003). 'I wouldn't want it on my CV or their records': Medical students' experiences of help-seeking for mental health problems. *Medical Education, 37*, 873–880.
Christakis, D., & Feudtner, C. (1997). Temporary matters: The ethical consequences of transient social relationships in medical training. *JAMA, 278*, 739–743.
Cooper, B. (2011). *Empathy in Education: Engagement, Values and Achievement*. London: Bloomsbury Publishing.
Costa, P., Alves, R., Neto, I., Marvao, P., Portela, M., & Costa, M. J. (2014). Associations between medical student empathy and personality: A Multi-institutional study. *PLoS ONE, 9*, e89254–e89254.

Coulehan, J., & Williams, P. (2003). Conflicting professional values in medical education. *Cambridge Quarterly of Healthcare Ethics, 12,* 7–20.
Cutler, J., Harding, K., Mozian, S., Wright, L. L., Pica, A. G., Masters, S., et al. (2009). Discrediting the notion "working with 'crazies' will make you 'crazy'": Addressing stigma and enhancing empathy in medical student education. *Advances in Health Sciences Education, 14,* 487–502.
Dyrbye, L. N., Thomas, M. R., & Shanafelt, T. D. (2005). Medical student distress: Causes, consequences and proposed solutions. *Mayo Clinic Proceedings, 80,* 1613–1622.
Dyrbye, L. N., Thomas, M. R., Power, D. V., Durning, S., Moutier, C., Massie, F. S., et al. (2010). Burnout and serious thoughts of dropping out of medical school: A multi-institutional study. *Academic Medicine, 85,* 94–102.
Eikeland, H. L., Ornes, K., Finset, A., & Pedersen, R. (2014). The physician's role and empathy—A qualitative study of third year medical students. *BMC Medical Education, 14,* 165–173.
Ekman, E., & Halpern, J. (2015). Professional distress and meaning in health care: Why professional empathy can help. *Social Work in Health Care, 54,* 633–650.
Epstein, R. M. (2014). Realizing Engel's biopsychosocial vision: Resilience, compassion, and quality of care. *The International Journal of Psychiatry in Medicine, 47,* 275–287.
Firth-Cozens, J. (2001). Medical student stress. *Medical Education, 35,* 6–7.
Frost, H. D., & Regehr, G. (2013). "I am a doctor": Negotiating the discourses of standardization and diversity in professional identity construction. *Academic Medicine, 88,* 1570–1577.
General Medical Council. (2009). *Tomorrow's Doctors: Outcomes and Standards for Undergraduate Medical Education*. London: General Medical Council.
General Medical Council. (2013). *Doctors' Use of Social Media*. London: General Medical Council.
Goldacre, M. J., Turner, G., & Lambert, T. W. (2004). Variation by medical school in career choices of UK graduates of 1999 and 2000. *Medical Education, 38,* 249–258.
Halpern, J. (2001). *From Detached Concern to Empathy: Humanizing Medical Practice*. Oxford: Oxford University Press.
Halpern, J. (2014). From idealized clinical empathy to empathic communication in medical care. *Medicine, Health Care and Philosophy, 17,* 301–311.

Hardy, C. (2017). Empathizing with patients: The role of interaction and narratives in providing better patient care. *Medicine, Healthcare and Philosophy.*, *20*, 237–248.

Harrison, R. L., & Westwood, M. J. (2009). Preventing vicarious traumatization of mental health therapists: Identifying protective practices. *Psychotherapy: Theory, Research, Practice, Training, 46*(2), 203–219.

Hinze, S. W. (1999). Gender and the body of medicine or at least some body parts: (Re) constructing the prestige hierarchy of medical specialties. *The Sociological Quarterly, 40*, 217–239.

Hojat, M., Zuckerman, M., Magee, M., Mangione, S., Nasca, T., Vergare, M., et al. (2005). Empathy in medical students as related to specialty interest, personality, and perceptions of mother and father. *Personality and Individual Differences, 39*, 1205–1215.

Jackson, V., Mack, J., Matsuyama, R., Lakoma, M. D., Sullivan, A. M., Arnold, R., et al. (2008). A qualitative study of oncologists' approaches to end-of-life care. *Journal of Palliative Medicine, 11*, 893–906.

Janssen, A. L., & Macleod, R. D. (2010). What can people approaching death teach us about how to care? *Patient Education and Counseling, 81*, 251–256.

Jennings, M. (2009). Medical student burnout: Interdisciplinary exploration and analysis. *Journal of Medical Humanities, 30*, 253–269.

Kang, J., Djafari Marbini, H., Patel, P., Fawcett, N., & Leaver, L. (2015). Survey of medical students' use of social media. *The Clinical Teacher, 12*, 373–377.

Karnieli-Miller, O., Vu, T. R., Frankel, R. M., Holtman, M. C., Clyman, S. G., Hui, S. L., et al. (2011). Which experiences in the hidden curriculum teach students about professionalism? *Academic Medicine, 86*, 369–377.

Kearney, M. K., Weininger, R. B., Vachon, M. L. S., Harrison, R. L., & Mount, B. M. (2009). Self-care of physicians caring for patients at the end of Life "being connected…. a key to survival". *JAMA, 301*, 1155–1164.

Kerasidou, A., & Horn, R. (2016). Making space for empathy: Supporting doctors in the emotional labour of clinical care. *BMC Medical Ethics, 17*, 8–13.

Konrath, S. H., O'Brien, E. H., & Hsing, C. (2010). Changes in dispositional empathy in American college students over time: A meta-analysis. *Personality and Social Psychology Review, 15*, 180–198.

Kozéki, B., & Berghammer, R. (1992). The role of empathy in the motivational structure of school children. *Personality and Individual Differences, 13*, 191–203.

Langewitz, W., Denz, M., Keller, A., Kiss, A., Rütimann, S., & Wössmer, B. (2002). Spontaneous talking time at start of consultation in outpatient clinic: Cohort study. *BMJ, 325,* 682–683.

Lempp, H., & Seale, C. (2004). The hidden curriculum in undergraduate medical education: Qualitative study of medical students' perceptions of teaching. *BMJ, 329,* 770–773.

Marcum, J. A. (2013). The role of empathy and wisdom in medical practice and pedagogy: Confronting the hidden curriculum. *Journal of Biomedical Education, 2013,* 1–8.

Marshall, G. R. E., & Hooker, C. (2016). Empathy and affect: What can empathied bodies do? *Medical Humanities, 42,* 128–134.

Marvel, M. K., Epstein, R. M., Flowers, K., & Beckman, H. B. (1999). Soliciting the patient's agenda: Have we improved? *JAMA, 281,* 283–287.

Mayes, C. (2009). Pastoral power and the confessing subject in patient-centred communication. *Journal of Bioethical Inquiry, 6,* 483–493.

Monrouxe, L. V., & Rees, C. E. (2012). "It's just a clash of cultures": Emotional talk within medical students' narratives of professionalism dilemmas. *Advances in Health Sciences Education, 17,* 671–701.

Monrouxe, L. V., Rees, C. E., Endacott, R., & Ternan, E. (2014). 'Even now it makes me angry': Health care students' professionalism dilemma narratives. *Medical Education, 48,* 502–517.

Neumann, M., Edelhaeuser, F., Tauschel, D., Fischer, M. R., Wirtz, M., Woopen, C., et al. (2011). Empathy decline and its reasons: A systematic review of studies with medical students and residents. *Academic Medicine, 86,* 996–1009.

Nogueira-Martins, M. C. F., Nogueira-Martins, L. A., & Turato, E. R. (2006). Medical students' perceptions of their learning about the doctor–patient relationship: A qualitative study. *Medical Education, 40,* 322–328.

Ozbay, F., Johnson, D. C., Dimoulas, E., Morgan III, C., Charney, D., & Southwick, S. (2007). Social support and resilience to stress: From neurobiology to clinical practice. *Psychiatry, 4*(5), 35.

Paro, H. M. S., Silveira, P. S. P., Perotta, B., Gannam, S., Enns, S. C., Giaxa, R. R. B., et al. (2014). Empathy among medical students: Is there a relation with quality of life and burnout? *PloS One, 9,* e94133–e94133.

Pickard, M., Bates, L., Dorian, M., Greig, H., & Saint, D. (2000). Alcohol and drug use in second-year medical students at the University of Leeds. *Medical Education, 34,* 148–150.

Ratanawongsa, N., Teherani, A., & Hauer, K. E. (2005). Third-year medical students' experiences with dying patients during the internal medicine clerkship: A qualitative study of the informal curriculum. *Academic Medicine, 80,* 641–647.

Reblin, M., & Uchino, B. N. (2008). Social and emotional support and its implication for health. *Current Opinion in Psychiatry, 21,* 201–205.

Rees, C. E., & Monrouxe, L. V. (2011). "A morning since eight of just pure grill": A multischool qualitative study of student abuse. *Academic Medicine, 86,* 1374–1382.

Rees, C. E., Monrouxe, L. V., & McDonald, L. A. (2013). Narrative, emotion and action: analysing 'most memorable' professionalism dilemmas. *Medical Education, 47,* 80–96.

Schweller, M., Ribeiro, D. L., Celeri, E. V., & de Carvalho-Filho, M. A. (2017). Nurturing virtues of the medical profession: Does it enhance medical students' empathy? *International Journal of Medical Education, 8*, 262.

Shanafelt, T., West, C., Zhao, X. H., Novotny, P., Kolars, J., Habermann, T., et al. (2005). Relationship between increased personal well-being and enhanced empathy among internal medicine residents. *Journal of General Internal Medicine, 20,* 559–564.

Tavakol, S., Dennick, R., & Tavakol, M. (2012). Medical students' understanding of empathy: A phenomenological study. *Medical Education, 46,* 306–316.

Thomas, M. R., Dyrbye, L. N., Huntington, J. L., Lawson, K., Novotny, P. J., Sloan, J. A., et al. (2007). How do distress and well-being relate to medical student empathy? A multicenter study. *Journal of General Internal Medicine, 22,* 177–183.

Timm, A. (2014). 'It would not be tolerated in any other profession except medicine': Survey reporting on undergraduates' exposure to bullying and harassment in their first placement year. *BMJ Open* [Online], 4. Available http://dx.doi.org/10.1136/bmjopen-2014-005140. Accessed January 29, 2018.

Twenge, J. M. (2013). The evidence for generation me and against generation we. *Emerging Adulthood, 1,* 11–16.

Verghese, A. (2008). Culture shock—Patient as icon, icon as patient. *New England Journal of Medicine, 359,* 2748–2751.

von Harscher, H., Desmarais, N., Dollinger, R., Grossman, S., & Aldana, S. (2018). The impact of empathy on burnout in medical students: New findings. *Psychology, Health & Medicine, 23,* 295–303.

Vossen, H. G., & Valkenburg, P. M. (2016). Do social media foster or curtail adolescents' empathy? A longitudinal study. *Computers in Human Behavior, 63,* 118–124.
Wear, D., Zarconi, J., Kumagai, A., & Cole-Kelly, K. (2014). Slow medical education. *Academic Medicine, 90,* 289–293.
Zenasni, F., Boujut, E., Woerner, A., & Sultan, S. (2012). Burnout and empathy in primary care: Three hypotheses. *British Journal of General Practice, 62,* 346–347.

7

Barriers to Empathy: The Curriculum

Overview

This chapter addresses the formal curriculum and its effects on empathy. The chapter begins with a discussion of whether empathy can be taught. The students describe a lack of teaching about empathy and the neglect of psychosocial aspects of the patient's situation. They talk about the strong biomedical bias in their teaching and its negative effect of empathy. Other factors such as negative role models, assessment and feedback are explored in relation to empathy in the student–patient relationship.

Can Empathy Be Taught?

Some students, who viewed empathy as an attribute, claimed that empathy could not be taught, but others argued that their empathy might be enhanced by teaching. Gina speculated that different dimensions of empathy might be amenable to teaching,

D. I. Jeffrey, *Exploring Empathy with Medical Students*,
https://doi.org/10.1007/978-3-030-11211-0_7

> I am sceptical about the extent to which teaching styles can change underlying empathy. (Marilyn, Year 2)

> It is the encouragement of it though, rather than, this is how to be empathetic. (Olive, Year 2)

> Maybe the idea of seeing it from their perspective maybe that can be taught. (Gina, Year 4)

Although some students were doubtful initially whether empathy could be taught, by the end of the course, some were convinced that teaching empathy was possible.

> many aspects of empathy can be taught. Yes, definitely, there are things that can be done. (Neville, Year 6)

The students' uncertainty as to whether empathy could be taught was reflected in the medical education literature (Wear and Zarconi 2008; Jeffrey and Downie 2016). However, most authors agreed that empathy can be influenced by education but were less certain whether any changes in empathy were sustained (Stepien and Baernstein 2006; Pedersen 2010; Batt-Rawden et al. 2013; Kelm et al. 2014; Kiosses et al. 2016; Georgi et al. 2014; Wündrich et al. 2017).

There has been a tendency in undergraduate medical education to present empathy in isolation, as something different from clinical understanding (Pedersen 2010; Shapiro 2008; Foster and Freeman 2008). Downie argued that empathy should not be taught, since feelings might impair sound clinical judgement. He maintained that a doctor's friendly manner was sufficient (Jeffrey and Downie 2016).

Stepien and Baernstein (2006) reviewed the literature describing interventions aimed to foster empathy. They identified thirteen studies which described initiatives to enhance empathy, nine reporting a quantitative increase in student empathy and six reporting a qualitative increase (two studies measured both quantitative and qualitative outcomes). They concluded that, despite methodological difficulties, educational interventions could increase medical student empathy (Stepien and Baernstein 2006). One limitation of the studies was that they did not consider that the students' ability to empathise might be affected by the clinical context. This weakness made it difficult to extrapolate these results to empathetic behaviour at the bedside (Stepien and Baernstein 2006). The authors suggested that future research should be directed at understanding the components of empathy that improve patient satisfaction, clinical outcomes and physician well-being (Stepien and Baernstein 2006). They suggested that such understanding might allow teachers to target their interventions on specific dimensions of empathy (Stepien and Baernstein 2006). Authors have suggested that medical schools need to attend to specific issues in the learning environment, such as those identified in this research, to encourage empathy (Dunham et al. 2017).

Batt-Rawden et al. (2013) systematically reviewed the literature, from 2004 to 2012, on educational interventions which claimed to enhance empathy. They found fifteen quantitative studies and three qualitative studies with common methodological flaws, namely: a lack of a control group, single institution studies and measurement of attitudes rather than skills (Batt-Rawden et al. 2013). Fifteen articles reported significant increases in empathy and the authors concluded that educational interventions could be effective in maintaining and enhancing empathy but were uncertain as to their long-term effects (Batt-Rawden et al. 2013). They recommended that medical educators should consider using relationship-centred care as a foundation for their interventions to teach empathy (Batt-Rawden et al. 2013). They also called for controlled longitudinal studies to research the reported decline in empathy of medical students (Batt-Rawden et al. 2013). This research addressed the call for a longitudinal qualitative study although it was not a 'controlled' study in the positivist sense. Two further comprehensive reviews of empathy development (Pedersen 2010; Kelm et al. 2014), also identified a number of interventions in medical education which attempted to enhance empathy in medical students including:

- patient narratives and the creative arts (Shapiro et al. 2004)
- reflective essays and point-of-view writing (Shapiro et al. 2006)

- personal illness narratives: using reflective writing (DasGupta and Charon 2004)
- drama (Lim et al. 2011)
- communication skills training (Shapiro et al. 2009; Bayne 2011)
- problem-based learning (PBL) (Karaoglu and Seker 2011)
- patient interviews (Mullen et al. 2010).

Recent research suggests that role play, Balint groups, simulation training, communication skills training and greater patient involvement are all initiatives which can improve students' empathy (Koblar et al. 2018; du Vaure et al. 2017; Plotkin and Shochet 2018; Pohontsch et al. 2018; Kataoka et al. 2018).

Jackson et al. (2015) adopted a different approach, rather than simply addressing interventions directed at the student, they suggested that enhancing empathetic consultations required attention to both the student and the patient. Recently there have been initiatives in the UK to enhance empathy in healthcare settings as a response to the perceived need to humanise medical care (Shea and Lionis 2014). One example is the online Connecting, Assessing, Responding and Empowering (CARE) approach developed at the University of Glasgow to enhance empathy in primary care staff (Bikker et al. 2012; Fitzgerald et al. 2014). In another innovative development, The Point of Care Foundation in the UK have adopted Schwartz Center rounds, developed in the USA, which bring together hospital staff to discuss emotional and psychological care of patients in a group setting (Goodrich 2012). Such facilitated group sessions with medical students might have a place in medical undergraduate education.

It appeared, from this review of educational interventions, that the consensus was that empathy could be enhanced or facilitated in a number of ways but as there were no long-term studies, it was not possible to see if these effects were sustained. It is probable that no single approach will be the solution but rather tailoring a variety of strategies to enhance empathy in medical students will be the most effective way of teaching empathy (Archer and Meyer 2018).

Lack of Teaching About Empathy

Several students commented that there was little teaching on empathy during their training. They suggested that the lack of emphasis on empathy was related to a lack of patient contact.

> I wouldn't say that much kind of formal or even informal kind of on this subject at the moment but I think that is because we haven't seen many patients yet. (Fiona, Year 1)

Connie wondered whether the lack of teaching on empathy was because the university assumed that medical students would be naturally empathetic.

> Empathy can get occasionally missed off and I think it is because take it for granted we are going to connect with patients. (Connie, Year 2)

Students noticed that their teachers placed more emphasis on their clinical skills and factual issues.

> It gets drilled into you some clinical facts but I don't think empathy is driven into us nearly enough. (Connie, Year 2)

They identified specific gaps in their teaching such as emotional regulation and empathising with minority groups.

> We have never had someone sit there and maybe talk about the idea of empathy as a concept or maybe sort of the boundaries in communication and how much you want to attach and invest in patients and how much is appropriate. [...] I think it would be something beneficial. (Gina, Year 4)
>
> LGBT on the other hand, again we don't get taught about it. (Olive, Year 3)

Students differentiated teaching on empathy from teaching of communication skills. They suggested that learning about empathy was something that was acquired after clinical experience with patients and from observing good practice.

> I don't think we have had formal teaching on it. I mean we have had clinical communication teaching but these are hard things to teach. […] they are skills and attributes you pick up as you go along. (Neville, Year 4)

> probably just by seeing, just experience with real patients and seeing other people and copying what they do […] I suppose it is not something really be taught, it is more something you learn by watching others. (Lisa, Year 4)

Fiona reflected on the problem of meeting the differing needs of students and the pressure on the curriculum which made teaching empathy in isolation a lower priority for the university.

> empathy teaching it comes very naturally to some people but some people it might be something they might need slightly more time on and also support [….] you can't get a class and split, […]. You can't do that so you have got to give the same teaching to everyone. (Fiona, Year 2)

Students claimed that they were not taught about empathy or about emotional regulation. Some students identified parts of the formal curriculum which attempted to teach them empathy as a separate topic but discussed the limitations of these approaches. They suggested that there were missed opportunities to introduce the paticnt's experience into their teaching. For instance, some students were sceptical of problem-based learning (PBL), as a way of teaching empathy, implying that discussion of the nuanced nature of empathy was overlooked. This sense that the university was missing chances to incorporate empathy into teaching was a common theme.

> I don't deny that PBL could be a good opportunity to think about empathy but I have not in my experience of PBL over the last year I have really barely had any discussions on empathy and on how the patient feels. (Connie, Year 2)

> We didn't do anything, for example, about how the patient would cope with this kind of thing. (Bill, Year 2)

Students also noticed that the patient's experience was often omitted from their lectures, which focused instead on the diagnosis and management of disease and sometimes promoted a defensive style of practice.

> I think what was strange he didn't mention anything about the patient's experience. (Bill, Year 2)

> we have had lots of lectures about covering your own back[...] I think people are worried about getting too emotionally involved. (Helen, Year 2)

However, when lectures did include the patient's experience, they did not appeal to every student. Some students, according to Olive, took longer to appreciate that medical education should be centred on the patient's experience rather than revising for exams.

> it was something poignant, it was something that half people you would speak to say 'Yeah that was really glad got to hear that', other half, 'Oh well we got this to be revising for and we have been taken out of here.' (Olive, Year 3)

Much of the students' communication skills training was with simulated, rather than real patients; many students referred to the artificial nature of these consultations. However, some students did find this method useful, provided they adopted the role.

> having an actor is better than nothing. At the same time, it is also a slightly false situation. (Paula, Year 4)

> I think you have to really get yourself in that frame of mind and some level convince yourself that is actually happening. (Olive, Year 2)

Other students implied that the formal communication courses did not develop their empathy, but seeing patients was more useful. Gina claimed that teaching empathy was more complex than the medical school acknowledged.

> we do have communication skills workshops we have sort have had the last year we have simulated patient. […] but I don't know how much of that actually influenced me. (Gina, Year 4)

Some students speculated whether communications skills training with simulated patients possibly encouraged them to develop a form of fake empathy. Gina argued that communication skills can be taught to help those who find it difficult to express themselves but saw genuine empathy as an attribute.

> everyone has varying degrees of how open they are and that is not a bad thing. That is why we teach communication skills, because you can portray yourself in a way that you behave and interaction that appears empathic even if you're not particularly, not that you are a cold bad person who doesn't feel anything. (Gina, Year 5)

Successful teaching requires an understanding of the students' needs, beliefs, values and learning styles (Roberts et al. 2012). Students described a lack of teaching of empathy, or opportunities to discuss the subject with experienced clinicians (Lempp and Seale 2004). They identified missed opportunities to involve the patient's experience in their teaching; in problem-based learning, lectures and group discussions. It was considered that communication skills training did not enhance empathy but risked the development of fake empathy. Such training usually involved simulated patient encounters, in which a trained lay person role-plays a patient (Underman 2015). Authors have pointed to the limitation of teaching empathy with simulated patients (Bleakley and Bligh 2008; Wear and Varley 2008). They have argued that there is a risk that if communication with the patient is taught simply as a skill to be acquired and assessed, then resulting relationships with patients may be shallow and mechanistic (Marshall and Bleakley 2009). However others have pointed out that if the students can imagine that the experience is real, such teaching gave them an opportunity to practise empathy in a safe environment (Underman 2015). However, allowing students to practise their communication skills with real patients does not mean that they should necessarily start with complex tasks, such as breaking bad news (Wear and Varley 2008). A tension exists between authenticity and artificiality, most of the students proposed that fake consultations generated fake empathy. It appears that both the simulated patient and the student put on a performance rather than empathising (Perrella 2016). If empathy cannot exist in this artificial environment, it casts doubt on the validity of assessing empathy in an OSCE situation with simulated patients (Perrella 2016).

A study of the effect of simulated consultations on medical students' empathy found that the debriefing after the research encounter gave the students an opportunity to discuss the student–patient relationship (Schweller et al. 2014). The authors concluded that it was this discussion, outside their research, that influenced students to become more empathetic with patients (Schweller et al. 2014). Wear and Varley (2008) suggested that true empathy was not a simulation, nor simply a competence, but a treasure to have and to receive, reflecting a transcendent quality to empathy.

Lack of Patient Contact

The students regretted their lack of patient contact in the first three years of their course.

> this university has very very little patient contact in the first two years so the fact we are seeing loads patients in the clinical years is normal. What is not normal is how few we saw for our first two years here. (Marilyn, Year 4)

> from first semester in first year we do meet these patients but there is absolutely no doubt that when you go from second year to new year four then that is the clinical change that happens. (Olive, Year 3)

The first-year students wanted more patient contact and argued that it was an effective way to develop empathy. Their limited patient contact was focused on taking an effective history and clinical examination rather dealing with emotions. They implied that their teaching encouraged them to view the patient as a resource for them to practise their clinical skills.

> it all seems to be about getting the most out of the patients rather than any this how you should feel like a deeper thing. (Olive, Year 1)

However, a few students had reservations about increasing the patient contact earlier in the course. Connie explained that she was more concerned with the scientific elements of the history rather than dealing with any psychosocial concerns of the patient.

> I was probably more preoccupied that I got everything they were saying written down or making sure that I had asked the right questions or that I understood conditions well enough. (Connie, Year 3)

Another theme which arose from the students' stories was their lack of exposure to patients from minority groups or different cultures. Some students suggested that perhaps cultural issues were ignored by their tutors for a fear of appearing racist. Helen suggested that this might explain the apparent reluctance of some tutors to help overseas students with their communication skills.

> They [lecturers] made a few jokes about religion and I suppose loads of people do that. (Bill, Year 3)

> I don't think we have ever discussed it. Discussed anyone being homeless. (Olive, Year 3)

> I think people are worried about coming across as being racist or anti or against the foreign student and foreign doctors they are scared to flag up. (Helen, Year 3)

> if she had been communicating in her native language she would have been fine with talking to patients. It was because of her unfamiliarity with nuance and body language and stuff in our language and that was reason. But obviously that can't be highlighted, as obviously that is not her fault. I think it is a catch- 22. (Helen, Year 3)

The students also described problems of continuity and in accessing patients on some wards which made empathising difficult.

> I think that is the difficulty with medical school curriculum as the rotations are so short and you might see a patient on the wards for a few days and follow their case through but for the most part you are just seeing a consultation with a patient. (Gina, Year 4)

> there are certain wards that have reputations for being OK to go to and others don't. (Paula, Year 4)

Students were aware of their lack of life experience and claimed that this challenged their empathy.

> it is difficult because we are only twenty year-old protected children and they have really long lives with lots dramatic things happening and we can never understand how that would be. (Ida, Year 4)

Sometimes language and cultural differences hampered an empathetic approach. For instance working through a translator could inhibit empathy.

> it is going to be more difficult to try and connect with the patient and try and understand normally for cultural reason but the language barrier is a mountain. (Neville, Year 5)

> certainly if they are speaking through a translator. I think it can be difficult to completely get across what they are feeling, what you are feeling. (Lisa, Year 4)

The students identified face-to-face contact with real patients as one of the most effective ways of enhancing empathy. They claimed that the minimal patient contact in the first three years was a lost opportunity to develop their empathy. These findings are supported by other studies (Lempp and Seale 2004; Ratanawongsa et al. 2005). In a study of students' preclinical experiences, the authors found a gap between theory and practice in the students' desire for patient contact

(Nogueira-Martins et al. 2006). In the same study, students described their teachers' lack of interest in psychosocial care as another factor which inhibited empathy (Nogueira-Martins et al. 2006). They noted that a lack of continuity of contact with patients risked the development of detachment (Montgomery 2006). In another study introducing empathy training in the first year the authors found that this early intervention was helpful (Plotkin and Shochet 2018).

Students identified a lack of exposure to patients from ethnic minority groups, different cultures and LGBT people. Wayne et al. (2011) suggested that treating patients from disadvantaged backgrounds was associated with students' negative attitudes and an intolerance of ambiguity. However, the students in this research wanted to engage with people from differing cultures and backgrounds. A study of cultural awareness in medical students, in the context of caring for refugees, also found that they were interested in cross-cultural communication (Griswold et al. 2007). Cutler et al. (2009) found medical students' interaction with patients with psychiatric problems could enhance their empathy. Millennial learners (students who turned 18 in the year 2000) are characterised as being accepting of diversity (Roberts et al. 2012).

Students in my research talked about patients who challenged their empathy reflecting the findings of another study which concluded that medical students found emotional issues were one of the most challenging aspects in their encounters with patients (Bower et al. 2009). Earlier research indicated that students appreciated having time with patients to establish empathy (Ratanawongsa et al. 2005; Cutler et al. 2009). In particular, they claimed that providing end-of-life care to patients was a powerful way of developing empathy (Ratanawongsa et al. 2005). Students found that consultations with difficult patients those with mental health problems and those in situations of conflict were challenging but helped to develop their empathy (Nogueira-Martins et al. 2006; Cutler et al. 2009; Tavakol et al. 2012; Eikeland et al. 2014). Students recognised a need to be accessible to patients in order to establish empathy (Nogueira-Martins et al. 2006). They found acting as a patient's advocate was helpful, and suggested that humility was related to empathy (Griswold et al. 2007; Eikeland et al. 2014). Storytelling was described by some students as an effective way to learn about empathy, echoing Charon's ideas for developing narrative competence (Griswold et al. 2007; Charon 2001).

To explore the effect of the patient experience in empathy, Wilkes and Hoffman (2002) conducted an observational study of nine second-year medical students who were admitted to hospital on three consecutive weekends for a day including an overnight stay. The key themes which emerged from their study were a sense of loss of privacy and observing that nurses took time to talk and listen to 'student-patients', in contrast, they experienced coldness from the doctors. The study found that the students' primary concern after their experience was to improve the human aspects of the patient experience (Wilkes et al. 2002).

Ideas, Concerns and Expectations (ICE)

Students described how their approach to taking a history was formulaic at first but later became more flexible. They noticed that the focus of history-taking was on asking questions rather than a more receptive empathetic approach.

> our teaching was more focussed on the questions you would ask the patient rather than the way you would interact the patient. (Neville, Year 4)

They reflected on becoming more adaptable in their approach to history-taking. At an early stage, their focus was on gathering the medical facts. In the clinical years, some students found they were having a conversation with the patient.

> I think that is a really important part of learning to take history at the beginning of the year and if you learn to do it well enough you quite happy to break away from it. (Kim, Year 4)

A part of the patient's history which is particularly concerned with empathy is exploring their point of view. They need to be asked about their ideas of what is happening to them, giving them an opportunity to talk about their concerns and expectations. 'Ideas, concerns and expectations' have been incorporated into formal teaching of history-taking by the acronym ICE. Students found it strange that were expected to add ICE on to the end of their consultation. It was considered as a separate entity and was assessed as such in the OSCE.

> ideas, concerns,expectations, is one the most interesting and most valuable part of the history, because you get an idea how they see it and that is almost like empathy. (Fiona, Year 3)

> We get marks for ICE and I think that has coloured people's view on it. [...] it has turned into something, Oh I must do ICE then I will get marks, and I think that is poor. (Fiona, Year 3)

Some students suggested ICE should inform the whole consultation not just the end, arguing that it could be difficult to be presented with demands from the patient at the end of the consultation.

> how is that helpful to get all that information just at the end? (Edward, Year 4)

On the other hand, Jenny liked a structured view of history-taking and saw ICE as something to include in exams. She admitted that she might not ask about ICE in clinical practice, if short of time.

> I do use it sometimes. I don't use it every time I talk to someone just because it takes an extra ten minutes. (Jenny, Year 4)

Many students referred to ICE as a tickbox exercise which had lost its significance for empathising. Olive summarised their views,

> I suppose it is an important thing that you do get patients' ideas, concerns and expectations. But we so often joke about it. [...] You don't think about the fact that concerns can actually be something really concerning to the patient, but actually they have taken three months to come into the GP surgery and they finally come in. Because this concern that has been keeping them up every night until they decided to book appointment, or expectation they might be able to go home that day

> and have some peace of mind that they don't have cancer. and these are such important things but because [they] teach us, tick off ideas will get a mark, expectations double mark. (Olive, Year 3)

Students at another medical school reported that empathy was taught by applying the ICE acronym to engage with patients (Light et al. 2018). They commented that their teaching seemed to reduce empathy to a communication skill (Light et al. 2018).

Students claimed that much of the teaching of empathy was also a tickbox exercise; focused on preparing for exams rather than addressing patients' concerns.

> very box ticky because they're preparing us for our exams. (Marilyn, Year 2)

> [on a] surgical ward round it is very much kind of ticking boxes, firing through, so sometimes I don't feel that there is that kind of connection or asking the patient kind of any of their opinions or anything. (Lisa, Year 4)

Taking a history is a skilled act which requires the capacity to empathise with the patient and then to recount her story in a medical narrative (Montgomery 2006, p. 50). Teaching students to be suspicious of anecdote is yet another mechanism for inhibiting the influence of emotions. The biomedical emphasis in the way students are taught to take a history is exemplified by the marginalisation of the acronym ICE; ideas, concerns and expectations.

Empathy involves engaging with the patients' ideas, concerns and expectations (ICE) of their illness and its treatment (Tate 2005). Students described how these areas of taking a history were relegated to the end of their consultation and sometimes omitted. The separation of information gathering from emotional issues in history-taking was a feature of another qualitative study (Ohm et al. 2013). It seemed to students that their clinical teachers were not interested in the details of the patient's experience which were not established markers of disease (Montgomery 2006). This further accentuated the biomedical model, relegating the psychosocial concerns to an optional add-on to the 'proper' history, and resulting in further distancing from the patient.

Negative Role Models

While students encountered good role models they were distressed to witness occasional poor practice where doctors did not empathise with patients. For example, Marilyn was shocked by the way a neurosurgeon discussed possible surgery with a patient with a history of poor mental health.

> this surgeon tells her she can drop dead at any minute and she needs to have surgery and that surgery has 10% chance of death. Without giving them any space to process, without making sure they are OK, handing them the paperwork, saying it all in the same tone as if he was ordering a latte from Starbucks. (Marilyn, Year 4)

Marilyn wondered if surgeons needed empathy and explained that perhaps certain personality types sought specialties which required less empathy.

> I think it is a self-selecting thing. People who really want to have long term relationships with patients, people who love patient contact, people who interested in giving comfort don't become surgeons. (Marilyn, Year 2)

Amy was distressed by bedside teaching where the patient was ignored and doubted whether this was acceptable to treat a patient in this way.

> a shock to the system when having bedside teaching. [...] most of the bedside teaching was spent around the end of the bed looking at the patient chart discussing about the patients results, referring to patient as 'HE' instead of speaking to the patient directly.[...]I felt really, hmm, bad about it. (Amy, Year 5)

Students identified negative role models, describing doctors who showed little regard for the psychosocial concerns of the patient, particularly on surgical ward rounds. They felt distressed for the patient but were unable to speak out. Hicks et al. (2001) found that 61% of students had witnessed a clinical teacher acting unethically. In another study, students who had witnessed unethical behaviour were more like to behave unethically themselves, and to believe that their ethical values deteriorated during training (Feudtner et al. 1994). Bombeke et al. (2011) found that when students encountered negative role models they also lost their focus on the patient. However, one student in the research, who had been humiliated by a consultant, said her experience had made her resolved not to behave in a similar fashion when she became a doctor. Students implied that they encountered more negative than positive role models. Shapiro (2011) also reported a lack of positive role models who incorporated emotions into medical education.

Negative role models may undermine the students' willingness to connect with patients (Schweller et al. 2017). Students were reported to be distressed by negative role models, doctors who appeared insensitive, and lacking an interest in patients' psychosocial concerns (Lempp and Seale 2004; Ratanawongsa et al. 2005; Nogueira-Martins et al. 2006). Students also highlighted the stressful effect of humiliation and bullying by poor role models, that they maintained, reduced their capacity for empathy (Lempp and Seale 2004). In the UK, an ethnography describing the clinical teaching of year 4 students in the University of Edinburgh medical school emphasised the significant impact of positive and negative role models on students learning (Atkinson 1976).

Biomedical Bias

There was a consensus amongst the students that the course had a strong scientific biomedical bias and that psychosocial issues were neglected. Students implied that the scientific bias started at recruitment where medical schools were rated for research rather than teaching.

> I think our course is very scientific and very traditional in the way they have premedical years and the medical years. [...] But yeah, scientific from the start. (Olive, Year 2)

There were lectures in first year on Health, Ethics and Society (HES), which focused on psychosocial issues. However, at this stage students had minimal contact with patients so found it difficult to appreciate the significance of their teaching.

> I remember at the time everyone […] would be, why are we doing this?, how this is going to help us when we are doctors? (Gina, Year 4)

> Why did we get all that teaching when it didn't make sense? (Neville, Year 6)

Students also argued that the lack of patient contact in the first three years put too much emphasis on biomedical science. They acknowledged that science was important, but suggested it was the balance with psychosocial aspects of care which was skewed.

> there is much focus on the science and probably maybe because medicine has to be such a knowledge base thing and you are supposed to base everything on research and [the] latest literature and it has to be cutting edge. […] It is almost as if they have completely left out anything to do with the actual patient. (Bill, Year 2)

Students suggested that the university wanted to produce academic doctors although it professed to create 'caring competent doctors'. They argued that the introduction of the compulsory honours intercalated science degree provided further evidence of the medical school's commitment to a scientific agenda.

> I think they will ideally love to produce doctors who are very research orientated definitely, but also efficient and patient centred. (Amy, Year 4)

> When the conversation how all the biological stuff has finished and all done with, then maybe give some quick consideration to what happens when they leave the hospital or leave GP surgery. […] things like empathising with patients, understanding their situation and really how this one consultation slots into the rest of their life. It just it gets pushed back whether intentionally or not, it gets pushed back. (Connie, Year 2)

> I think they[medical educators] go 'first of all here is the problem this is how you sort it out', then they will consider, 'and by the way there are emotional aspects to this.' (Paula, Year 5)

Fiona, on the other hand, had a different perspective and said that she felt more confident in knowing some of the basic science before meeting people.

> I personally like knowing a bit more before I actually meet people. (Fiona, Year 2)

Other students like Diana and Amy thought the scientific agenda was also exemplified by the many evidence-based guidelines. Diana described the way surgeons are driven by these guidelines and suggested this may inhibit discussion. Amy wondered whether one reason why some treatments were continued inappropriately in dying patients was because doctors slavishly followed guidelines.

> there aren't many things we actually have to make the proper decision it is the right thing to do, there is NICE guideline for everything, so just have to go down that route. (Diana, Year 4)

> I think a lot is just so many guidelines and you just are just follow step one, step two, step three, step four. You don't' think so much [about the] patient anymore just think in terms of guidelines. And that is how we are taught in medical school as well, to follow guidelines. (Amy, Year 5)

It appeared that even in the clinical attachments the emphasis of teaching was on symptoms and signs rather than the psychological needs of the patient. Paula admitted that she would feel awkward raising emotional issues in a tutorial as it might be seen as a sign of weakness and suggested that the attention to psychological factors was tokenistic.

> Even innocuous things like oh there is a good murmur on the ward, everyone go listen to the murmur. (Gina, Year 6)

> that would almost be feel out of place actually to start talking in tutorials how do personally feel like you are. I don't know, it is a sign of weakness. (Paula, Year 4)

> they just throw an essay at you occasionally, and that is how addressing that you have done it[psychosocial care]. (Paula, Year 6)

Other students described being distressed by the biomedical bias of the curriculum. For example, Amy decided not to undertake an intercalated science degree as she felt she was losing her motivation to be a doctor during the preclinical years.

> A large part of me decided against intercalating because the first years dried me up a bit and I thought if I go out for a third year intercalating and science and whatever I might actually lose touch with medicine. (Amy, Year 4)

Paula claimed that the emphasis on the biomedical paradigm was present throughout the curriculum. She claimed that she had never received feedback from her tutors on how she related to a patient. Gina described NHS hospital medicine as dehumanising and was surprised by the numbers of patients who appeared uninformed about their condition.

> they are much more interested, Did you hear that? Or, Did you find that? [...]. I haven't had feedback how I related to a patient. (Paula, Year 5)

> the amount of people I have come across who really have no idea why they are there and what is happening. (Gina, Year 6)

> it seems like this intrinsic thing, remembering these are people, is almost lost, just through the way everything is organised. (Gina, Year 6)

Gina wondered if the biomedical bias would ever change, reflecting on the demographic differences which existed between patients and their doctors. She also commented on the curriculum changes which made the course even more scientific and competitive.

> It's so difficult because that kind of thinking and approach needs to come from the top down. So if it is not coming through medical curriculums how is it ever going to really change? (Gina, Year 6)

> changes to curriculum they are moving towards research excellence we produce research excellence. Who is going to get the most publication and be a highly published alumni? (Gina, Year 6)

Students have described their relational view of empathy with an emphasis on emotional connection. They were concerned that they were taught professionalism as a form of detachment from the patient.

The students described an emphasis in their teaching on the biomedical, or scientific, aspects of medicine, to the detriment of addressing the psychosocial aspects of patient care. The dichotomy between the biomedical and psychosocial was found in other studies (Pedersen 2010; Michalec 2011; Tavakol et al. 2012; Eikeland et al. 2014).

Forty years ago, the problems of a reductionist positivist view in medical practice and its resultant disease-orientated, biomedical model were identified by Engel (1978). He proposed a change to a patient-orientated biopsychosocial model of medical care which included psychosocial issues as well as the purely scientific (Engel 1978). Bloom (1989) also argued that academic scientific medicine paid tokenistic regard to the humanities in medical education. Montgomery developed these arguments by acknowledging the benefits of biomedicine, but proposed that clinical medicine be seen as an interpretative practice rather than as a science (Montgomery 2006, p. 5).

The students' stories showed that the biomedical model persisted in this curriculum, neglecting psychosocial aspects of care (Montgomery 2006; Epstein 2014). Lectures on psychosocial care were delivered in the first year, when the students, with little patient contact, could not fully appreciate their importance. They also found that the lack of patient contact in the first two years of the course combined with a compulsion to take an intercalated science degree in the third year further emphasised this university's commitment to scientific academic medicine and the development of a 'biomedical gaze' (Pedersen 2010).

This scientific stance reflected the dominant discourse where medicine became concerned largely with giving objective advice rather than connecting with the patient (Hardy 2017). Hardy (2017) warned that the suppression of empathy may become seen as a desirable skill for a physician. Such physicians, who embody this scientific attitude, can be role models for students who then risk losing empathy with patients (Hardy 2017). It seems, therefore, that adopting the scientific biomedical model exclusively can contribute to detachment and a lack of empathy.

Students reflected this dichotomy between the biomedical and psychosocial approaches. It appeared to them that the patient's experience seemed to be added on at the end of lectures in a tokenistic fashion, if it was addressed at all. Students described how, during ward rounds, clinicians appeared to be concerned with symptoms and signs rather than the psychological needs of patients. These findings resonated with other studies where students reflected on medicine's tendency to objectify patients, 'lumping' them into disease categories. Students realised they often lost sight of the uniqueness of the individual and identified a clinical environment focused on efficiency (Head et al. 2012; Wear and Zarconi 2008).

Other qualitative studies have also found that students learned that empathy was not as important as biomedical learning and the technical aspects of treatment (Eikeland et al. 2014; Ratanawongsa et al. 2005). The students in these studies talked about the emphasis in their teaching on a need to be objective and detached from the patient (Eikeland et al. 2014; Ratanawongsa et al. 2005). In some studies students, like those in this research, commented that evidence-based guidelines also were a mechanism for emphasising the scientific aspects of medicine rather than the patient's experience (Eikeland et al. 2014; Michalec 2011). Eikeland et al. (2014) suggested that a strong emphasis on scientific facts might alienate students from their own feelings, undermining opportunities for reflection. Montgomery however argued that evidence-based medicine needed to be incorporated with clinical experience in the practice of clinical judgement (Montgomery 2006).

In my research, the biomedical emphasis in the curriculum seemed to have two main effects on the students:

- It caused the students distress by neglecting psychosocial aspects of the patient's suffering which some authors have described as dehumanising (Sheikh et al. 2013).
- It resulted in them appearing distanced from patients who were sometimes seen as objects of intellectual interest.

Since the main focus of their medical educators was the students' knowledge base, they lacked adequate feedback on their empathy. Without this feedback, students in another study assumed empathy was of lesser importance to the medical school than biomedical aspects (Michalec 2011). Previous qualitative research found that students learned that empathy was not valued as much as biomedical learning and the technical aspects of treatment (Michalec 2011; Tavakol et al. 2012; Eikeland et al. 2014). The students were reported to have talked about an emphasis on clinical objectivity that implied a need to be detached from patients, since emotions were perceived to threaten rationality (Ratanawongsa et al. 2005; Eikeland et al. 2014). Some students expressed negative feelings about seeking the patients' views in case this provoked their emotions (Ratanawongsa et al. 2005). They described a strong emphasis on evidence-based medicine (EBM) and their need to absorb facts (Michalec 2011; Eikeland et al. 2014). Some were reported to have experienced a gap between theory and practice in relation to the medical school's attitude to psychosocial care, creating an uncomfortable dissonance for the students (Nogueira-Martins et al. 2006).

Medicine's identification with science appeared to offer students and doctors a way of avoiding emotions and their implicit danger of subjectivity (Montgomery 2006). The biomedical emphasis, in excluding psychosocial elements of care, promoted objectivity and detachment from patients (Halpern 2001; Pedersen 2010). However, there was a minority of students who welcomed the biomedical emphasis in this curriculum, which they claimed gave them more confidence when they came into contact with patients in year four. They acknowledged that both the biomedical and psychosocial elements were necessary for effective patient care but claimed that the balance between them was not appropriate in their course. Some students were not hopeful of the university redressing this imbalance, particularly in view of the recent change to make the intercalated science year compulsory.

Group Effects

The students described feeling self-conscious when they demonstrated empathy with a patient in front of their peer group. Helen said it was easier to share vulnerability with a patient in a one-to-one situation rather than in a group. She also suggested that males are affected more than females by the inhibiting effect of showing empathy in front of one's peers. Other students avoided emotional issues when they were in a group.

> in order to empathise with patients you have to expose your own vulnerability a little bit and that can that can feel like a scary thing to do in front of people you know. (Helen, Year 3)

> I think the group thing affects boys more than it does girls. I think for whatever sort of social reason it seems more almost socially acceptable for girls to show emotions than boys. (Helen, Year 3)

Kim described the problem of demonstrating empathy in front of consultants. Being watched did not prevent her feeling for the patient but it did inhibit her demonstration of that feeling. She further suggested that the patient also may have felt inhibited and unable to express her concerns.

> because you have people watching you and it makes you very much more aware of your body language, it doesn't' necessarily influence the thoughts that are going through your head. I think it maybe influences the rapport you can build with that patient if there were several people in the room. That obviously influences how much the patient opens up to you and what you gain from the consultation. Then that influences maybe your idea what the patient's thinking and feeling. (Kim, Year 4)

> They [consultants] are judging you on how quickly and concisely you can take a history. (Kim, Year 4)

Ida said that she avoided emotional issues in front of a group to protect the patient. Though she had empathy for the patient she felt that she was unable to show these feelings.

> But if there are a lot of other people around and I know that the other students are impatient to hear history and I probably wouldn't spend a long time exploring feelings of the patients. And also I wouldn't want to put the patient into the position having to talk about their feelings in front of so many people. (Ida, Year 6)

Assessment

Students described assessment as causing them stress which diminished their empathy. The medical school had a strong emphasis on assessment. From the start of their course, students were made aware that their marks counted towards their final grade and affected their career prospects. This generated a competitive stressful culture.

> So they break that down for every exam and every essay. So I suppose maybe the idea you can feel where you are in the year. (Bill, Year 3)

> when it comes to assessments you just end up preoccupied. Am I doing the right thing? not necessarily, am I getting better at knowing the person in front of me? (Connie, Year 3)

Bill recounted that when he was being assessed he disengaged from the patient because he was aware the judgement might affect his future. Connie found she could forget that she was being watched once her focus was on the patient rather than on her performance. She implied practice was crucial in relieving the stress of assessment.

> I wasn't interacting with the patient as a doctor-patient interaction in an informal way. (Bill, Year 3)

> actually once to get into it once you have focus on your patient you focus on their condition you sort of forget that you are being examined you forget someone is watching and critiquing you. (Connie, Year 3)

Students had a range of views as to whether the medical school assessed empathy. Lisa implied that empathy was not assessed by the medical school, and suggested that there ought to be some assessment of empathy. On the other hand, Paula claimed that empathy was assessed in their exams. Some students assumed that because empathy was not given many marks that it was not considered as important as having factual knowledge.

> You are not really getting marked on your empathetic approach to the patients so perhaps get pushed to the side during OSCEs. (Lisa, Year 4)

> I do get the impression [it's] what they look for in exams as well. (Paula, Year 6)

> The exams really mostly focus on clinical knowledge. Do you know this? Do you know that? and empathy seems to be, I don't know, a couple marks that I mean, sure important, there are marks for it. It does not give impression that it is that important. (Connie, Year 2)

Amy suggested that the OSCEs encouraged a fake empathy. Kim claimed that OSCEs were not an effective way of assessing their empathy, because of the shortage of time.

> I guess in OSCE you are kind of trained to just OK, cut to the chase, just ask the questions you are supposed to ask and then ticks and that is it. (Amy, Year 4)

> they try sometimes assess your empathy towards a patient. But I think it can be difficult to demonstrate it in an OSCE you have a clock sitting here with the time on it. (Kim, Year 4)

Students described difficulties in showing empathy in a group setting. This was because of embarrassment in raising emotional issues in front of others but was also motivated by protective feelings for the patient. It is possible that if bedside clinical teaching is conducted in small groups that students may appear to lack empathy when they are in fact experiencing emotional concern for the patient (Elder and Verghese 2015).

Feedback

Students maintained that there was a lack of helpful feedback from the medical school. Helen described a lack of encouragement and unsatisfactory feedback, which she suggested contributed to a competitive culture.

> You work and work for these exams and then nine out of ten times the feedback is not out in time or your results are not out in time which is a big kick in the teeth. (Helen, Year 3)

> You never get feedback personal feedback about areas of medicine you[have] done well in or areas that you can. All you get encourages [you] to compare yourself to other people, because all you get is your exam result and where that is on the bar graph or on the curve. (Helen, Year 3)

Some students suggested that their feedback to the university did not result in change. Others admitted that they would be fearful of giving the university honest feedback, because of their concerns about confidentiality.

> when you speak to other students in previous years who are older than us then it doesn't seem not much has changed. Or it doesn't really seem taken into consideration. (Bill, Year 3)

> it is quite difficult to give honest feedback and you are not entirely sure who is going to and where it is going. (Kim, Year 6)

Students remarked on the emphasis on assessment within the medical school and claimed this had the unwanted effects of encouraging competition and diminishing empathy. They perceived that the focus of assessment was on their factual knowledge rather than on their empathy. This emphasis was aggravated by a lack of feedback from their tutors on their empathetic skills, leaving them with the option of comparing themselves to their peers so promoting the competitive culture. Paradoxically, despite wanting feedback, students described how they were fearful to give the medical school their views because of a perceived lack of confidentiality.

Key Points

- The students identified a lack of emphasis on empathy in their teaching.
- Students wanted more patient contact and identified missed opportunities in their curriculum to include the patient experience.
- They described a tickbox approaches to teaching psychosocial care.
- They highlighted the inhibiting effect on their empathy of both negative role models and the strong biomedical emphasis of their teaching.
- The strong emphasis on assessment within the medical school created a barrier to empathy.

References

Archer, E., & Meyer, I. (2018). Teaching empathy to undergraduate medical students: 'One glove does not fit all'. *Medical Education,* 52, 1191.

Atkinson, P. (1976). *The Clinical Experience: An Ethnography of Medical Education* (PhD.). Durham University.

Batt-Rawden, S., Chisolm, M. S., Anton, B., & Flickinger, T. E. (2013). Teaching empathy to medical students: An updated, systematic review. *Academic Medicine, 88,* 1171–1177.

Bayne, H. B. (2011). Training medical students in empathic communication. *The Journal for Specialists in Group Work, 36,* 316–329.

Bikker, A. P., Mercer, S. W., & Cotton, P. (2012). Connecting, assessing, responding and empowering (CARE): A universal approach to person-centred, empathic healthcare encounters. *Education for Primary Care, 23,* 454–457.

Bleakley, A., & Bligh, J. (2008). Students learning from patients: Let's get real in medical education. *Advances in Health Sciences Education, 13,* 89–107.

Bloom, S. (1989). The medical school as a social organization: The sources of resistance to change. *Medical Education, 23,* 228–241.

Bombeke, K., Van Roosbroeck, S., De Winter, B., Debaene, L., Schol, S., Van Hal, G., et al. (2011). Medical students trained in communication skills show a decline in patient-centred attitudes: An observational study

comparing two cohorts during clinical clerkships. *Patient Education and Counseling, 84,* 310–318.
Bower, D. J., Young, S., Larson, G., Simpson, D., Tipnis, S., Begaz, T., et al. (2009). Characteristics of patient encounters that challenge medical students' provision of patient-centered care. *Academic Medicine, 84,* 74–78.
Charon, R. (2001). Narrative medicine—A model for empathy, reflection, profession, and trust. *JAMA, 286,* 1897–1902.
Cutler, J., Harding, K., Mozian, S., Wright, L. L., Pica, A. G., Masters, S., et al. (2009). Discrediting the notion "working with 'crazies' will make you 'crazy'": Addressing stigma and enhancing empathy in medical student education. *Advances in Health Sciences Education, 14,* 487–502.
DasGupta, S., & Charon, R. (2004). Personal illness narratives: Using reflective writing to teach empathy. *Academic Medicine, 79,* 351–356.
du Vaure, C. B., Lemogne, C., Bunge, L., Catu-Pinault, A., Hoertel, N., Ghasarossian, C., et al. (2017). Promoting empathy among medical students: A two-site randomized controlled study. *Journal of Psychosomatic Research, 103,* 102–107.
Dunham, L., Dekhtyar, M., Gruener, G., Cichoskikelly, E., Deitz, J., Elliott, D., et al. (2017). Medical student perceptions of the learning environment in medical school change as students transition to clinical training in undergraduate medical school. *Teaching and Learning in Medicine, 29,* 383–391.
Eikeland, H. L., Ornes, K., Finset, A., & Pedersen, R. (2014). The physician's role and empathy—A qualitative study of third year medical students. *BMC Medical Education, 14,* 165–173.
Elder, A., & Verghese, A. (2015). Bedside matters—Putting the patient at the centre of teaching and learning. *Journal of the Royal College of Physicians of Edinburgh, 45,* 186–187.
Engel, G. L. (1978). The biopsychosocial model and the education of health professionals. *Annals of the New York Academy of Sciences, 310,* 169–181.
Epstein, R. M. (2014). Realizing Engel's biopsychosocial vision: Resilience, compassion, and quality of care. *The International Journal of Psychiatry in Medicine, 47,* 275–287.
Feudtner, C., Christakis, D. A., & Christakis, N. A. (1994). Do clinical clerks suffer ethical erosion? Students' perceptions of their ethical environment and personal development. *Academic Medicine, 69,* 670–679.
Fitzgerald, N. M., Heywood, S., Bikker, A. P., & Mercer, S. W. (2014). Enhancing empathy in healthcare: Mixed-method evaluation of a pilot project implementing the CARE Approach in primary and community care settings in Scotland. *Journal of Compassionate Health Care, 1,* 1.

Foster, W., & Freeman, E. (2008). Poetry in general practice education: Perceptions of learners. *Family Practice, 25,* 294–303.

Georgi, E., Petermann, F., & Schipper, M. (2014). Are empathic abilities learnable? Implications for social neuroscientific research from psychometric assessments. *Social Neuroscience, 9,* 74–81.

Goodrich, J. (2012). Supporting hospital staff to provide compassionate care: Do Schwartz Center Rounds work in English hospitals? *Journal of the Royal Society of Medicine, 105,* 117–122.

Griswold, K., Zayas, L., Kernan, J. B., & Wagner, C. M. (2007). Cultural awareness through medical student and refugee patient encounters. *Journal of Immigrant and Minority Health, 9,* 55–60.

Halpern, J. (2001). *From Detached Concern to Empathy: Humanizing Medical Practice.* Oxford: Oxford University Press.

Hardy, C. (2017). Empathizing with patients: The role of interaction and narratives in providing better patient care. *Medicine, Healthcare and Philosophy, 20,* 237–248.

Head, B. A., Earnshaw, L. A., Greenberg, R. B., Morehead, R. C., Pfeifer, M. P., & Shaw, M. A. (2012). "I will never forget": What we learned from medical student reflections on a palliative care experience. *Journal of Palliative Medicine, 15,* 535–541.

Hicks, L. K., Lin, Y., Robertson, D. W., Robinson, D. L., & Woodrow, S. I. (2001). Understanding the clinical dilemmas that shape medical students' ethical development: Questionnaire survey and focus group study. *BMJ, 322,* 709–710.

Jackson, P., Eugène, F., & Tremblay, M.-P. B. (2015). Improving empathy in the care of pain patients. *AJOB Neuroscience, 6,* 25–33.

Jeffrey, D., & Downie, R. (2016). Empathy—Can it be taught? *Journal of the Royal College of Physicians of Edinburgh, 46,* 107–112.

Karaoglu, N., & Seker, M. (2011). Looking for winds of change with a PBL scenario about communication and empathy. *Healthmed, 5,* 515–521.

Kataoka, H., Iwase, T., Ogawa, H., Mahmood, S., Sato, M., Desantis, J., et al. (2018). Can communication skills training improve empathy? A six-year longitudinal study of medical students in Japan. *Medical Teacher*, 1–6. https// doi.org/10.1080/0142159X.2018.1460657. Accessed December 23, 2018.

Kelm, Z., Womer, J., Walter, J., & Feudtner, C. (2014). Interventions to cultivate physician empathy: A systematic review. *BMC Medical Education, 14,* 219–230.

Kiosses, V. N., Karathanos, V. T., & Tatsioni, A. (2016). Empathy promoting interventions for health professionals: A systematic review of RCTs. *Journal of Compassionate Health Care, 3,* 7–29.

Koblar, S., Cranwell, M., Koblar, S., Carnell, B., & Galletly, C. (2018). Developing empathy: Does experience through simulation improve medical-student empathy? *Medical Science Educator, 28,* 31–36.
Lempp, H., & Seale, C. (2004). The hidden curriculum in undergraduate medical education: Qualitative study of medical students' perceptions of teaching. *BMJ, 329,* 770–773.
Light, A., Gupta, T., Burrows, A., Nandakumar, M., Daniel, A., & Karthikeyan, S. (2018). Learning empathy: The medical student perspective. *The Clinical Teacher.* https://doi.org/101111/tct12801. Accessed December 23, 2018.
Lim, B., Moriarty, H., & Huthwaite, M. (2011). "Being-in-role": A teaching innovation to enhance empathic communication skills in medical students. *Medical Teacher, 33,* 663–669.
Marshall, R., & Bleakley, A. (2009). The death of Hector: Pity in Homer, empathy in medical education. *Medical Humanities, 35,* 7–12.
Michalec, B. (2011). Learning to cure, but learning to care? *Advances in Health Sciences Education, 16,* 109–130.
Montgomery, K. (2006). *How Doctors Think: Clinical Judgment and the Practice of Medicine.* Oxford: Oxford University Press.
Mullen, K., Nicolson, M., & Cotton, P. (2010). Improving medical students' attitudes towards the chronic sick: A role for social science research. *BMC Medical Education, 10,* 84–91.
Nogueira-Martins, M. C. F., Nogueira-Martins, L. A., & Turato, E. R. (2006). Medical students' perceptions of their learning about the doctor–patient relationship: A qualitative study. *Medical Education, 40,* 322–328.
Ohm, F., Vogel, D., Sehner, S., Wijnen-Meijer, M., & Harendza, S. (2013). Details acquired from medical history and patients' experience of empathy—Two sides of the same coin. *BMC Medical Education, 13,* 67–74.
Pedersen, R. (2010). Empathy development in medical education—A critical review. *Medical Teacher, 32,* 593–600.
Perrella, A. (2016). Fool me once: The illusion of empathy in interactions with standardized patients. *Medical Teacher, 38,* 1285–1287.
Plotkin, J. B., & Shochet, R. (2018). Beyond words: What can help first year medical students practice effective empathic communication? *Patient Education and Counseling, 101,* 2005–2010.
Pohontsch, N., Stark, A., Ehrhardt, M., Kötter, T., & Scherer, M. (2018). Influences on students' empathy in medical education: An exploratory interview study with medical students in their third and last year. *BMC Medical Education, 18,* 231.

Ratanawongsa, N., Teherani, A., & Hauer, K. E. (2005). Third-year medical students' experiences with dying patients during the internal medicine clerkship: A qualitative study of the informal curriculum. *Academic Medicine, 80,* 641–647.

Roberts, D. H., Newman, L. R., & Schwartzstein, R. M. (2012). Twelve tips for facilitating Millennials' learning. *Medical Teacher, 34,* 274–278.

Schweller, M., Costa, F. O., Antônio, M. Â. R., Amaral, E. M., & De Carvalho-Filho, M. A. (2014). The impact of simulated medical consultations on the empathy levels of students at one medical school. *Academic Medicine, 89,* 632–637.

Schweller, M., Ribeiro, D. L., Celeri, E. V., & De Carvalho-Filho, M. A. (2017). Nurturing virtues of the medical profession: Does it enhance medical students' empathy? *International Journal of Medical Education, 8,* 262.

Shapiro, J. (2008). Walking a mile in their patients' shoes: Empathy and othering in medical students' education. *Philosophy, Ethics, and Humanities in Medicine, 3,* 10–21.

Shapiro, J. (2011). Perspective: Does medical education promote professional alexithymia? A call for attending to the emotions of patients and self in medical training. *Academic Medicine, 86,* 326–332.

Shapiro, J., Morrison, E., & Boker, J. (2004). Teaching empathy to first year medical students: Evaluation of an elective literature and medicine course. *Education for Health, 17,* 73–84.

Shapiro, J., Rucker, L., Boker, J., & Lie, D. (2006). Point-of-view writing: A method for increasing medical students' empathy, identification and expression of emotion, and insight. *Education for Health: Change in Learning and Practice, 19,* 96–105.

Shapiro, S. M., Lancee, W. J., & Richards-Bentley, C. M. (2009). Evaluation of a communication skills program for first-year medical students at the University of Toronto. *BMC Medical Education, 9,* 11.

Shea, S., & Lionis, C. (2014). Introducing the Journal of Compassionate Health Care. *Journal of Compassionate Health Care, 1,* 7.

Sheikh, H., Carpenter, J., & Wee, J. (2013). Medical student reporting of factors affecting pre-clerkship changes in empathy: A qualitative study. *Canadian Medical Education Journal, 4,* e26–e34.

Stepien, K. A., & Baernstein, A. (2006). Educating for empathy—A review. *Journal of General Internal Medicine, 21,* 524–530.

Tate, P. (2005). Ideas, concerns and expectations. *Medicine, 33,* 26–27.

Tavakol, S., Dennick, R., & Tavakol, M. (2012). Medical students' understanding of empathy: A phenomenological study. *Medical Education, 46,* 306–316.

Underman, K. (2015). Playing doctor: Simulation in medical school as affective practice. *Social Science and Medicine, 136,* 180–188.

Wayne, S., Dellmore, D., Serna, L., Jerabek, R., Timm, C., & Kalishman, S. (2011). The association between intolerance of ambiguity and decline in medical students' attitudes toward the underserved. *Academic Medicine, 86,* 877–882.

Wear, D., & Varley, J. D. (2008). Rituals of verification: The role of simulation in developing and evaluating empathic communication. *Patient Education and Counseling, 71,* 153–156.

Wear, D., & Zarconi, J. (2008). Can compassion be taught? Let's ask our students. *Journal of General Internal Medicine, 23,* 948–953.

Wilkes, M., & Hoffman, J. (2002). Students benefit from experience of hospitalization. *Medical Education, 36,* 586–587.

Wilkes, M., Milgrom, E., & Hoffman, J. R. (2002). Towards more empathic medical students: A medical student hospitalization experience. *Medical Education, 36,* 528–533.

Wündrich, M., Schwartz, C., Feige, B., Lemper, D., Nissen, C., & Voderholzer, U. (2017). Empathy training in medical students—A randomized controlled trial. *Medical Teacher, 39,* 1096–1098.

8

Changes in Students' Empathy During Their Training

Overview

This book challenges the widely accepted view that students' empathy declines during their training. Students describe an increasing focus on the patient, distress at examples of a lack of empathy with patients and a concern that they remain empathetic doctors in the future. They also describe the ways in which they hide expression of their empathy in the interests of appearing 'efficient'.

Medical education is an initiation into a practice which involves the whole student, their attitudes, values, beliefs, behaviour, emotions and ideas (Montgomery 2006, p. 167). Some authors have described the process of professional socialisation as one of osmosis, a passive absorption of the culture of the medical school and a shaping of the self to gain a professional identity (Montgomery 2006). I explored students' professional socialisation within a range of experiences. For some students, professional socialisation might involve the adoption of a different world view and emotional orientations, a process which Monrouxe (2010) called 'identity dissonance'.

D. I. Jeffrey, *Exploring Empathy with Medical Students*,
https://doi.org/10.1007/978-3-030-11211-0_8

The 'Empathy Decline'

In contrast to the phenomenological approach adopted in this research, most studies of empathy in medical students have used a quantitative methodology. By conceptualising empathy as a personal attribute, they disregard relational and contextual aspects of empathy.

Three systematic reviews have reported instruments available to measure empathy and presented evidence for their reliability and validity (Hemmerdinger et al. 2007; Pedersen 2009; Sulzer et al. 2016). Hemmerdinger et al. (2007) found 50 relevant papers describing 36 different instruments of empathy measurement; however, only eight demonstrated evidence of reliability and validity. Only one, the Consultation and Relational Empathy (CARE) scale was considered a useful measure of empathy from the patient's perspective. It has been used as a tool for assessing the patient's perception of empathy in primary care (Hemmerdinger et al. 2007; Mercer et al. 2004, 2005; Price et al. 2006). Although the inclusion of the patient's voice in an assessment of empathy is to be welcomed, the CARE measure is founded on a presumption of empathy as a property of the doctor alone. There is no acknowledgement that a consultation with low empathy rating might be due to the fact that the patient was withdrawn or the context challenging (Alnoman 2014; Howick et al. 2017).

In Pedersen's extensive review of 206 publications of empathy research in medicine, 171 related to quantitative methods and only 33 explored empathy through qualitative methods (Pedersen 2009). He concluded that since self-reports may not correspond with empathy in practice, it should not be studied solely through quantitative approaches (Pedersen 2009).

In a recent systematic review of 109 quantitative studies, Sulzer et al. (2016) found that 20% of studies failed to define empathy, and only 13% used the definition they provided in the study. The authors concluded that there was a need for greater understanding of the mechanisms that shape empathy (Sulzer et al. 2016).

Empathy has been most frequently studied in medical practice through the Jefferson Scale of Physician Empathy (JSPE) and the Jefferson Scale of Empathy-Student Version (JSE-S). These scales explore attitudes of medical students or doctors, using a self-assessment questionnaire, outside the clinical setting (Hojat et al. 2001). The questionnaire consists of twenty items on a seven-point Likert scale. The JSPE originally was not intended to explore the philosophical dimensions of empathy, nor the processes of empathising, but was intended as an approximate indicator of empathy (Hojat et al. 2001).

There are limitations to studying empathy by this method. Measurement of empathy by self-assessment can generate inconsistencies due to a social desirability bias which might exist in medical students who wish to appear to be caring (Austin et al. 2007; Glaser et al. 2007). Although some correlations between self-reported and observed empathy have been shown, there have been conflicting results in using differing methods of assessing empathy. For example, a study showed self-assessed empathy, measured by the JSPE, decreased during the second and third years of the undergraduate course, whereas observed empathy during an objective structured clinical examination (OSCE) increased during the same period (Chen et al. 2010). Berg et al. (2011) found that there was no conclusive association between empathy score measured by the JSPE and simulated patients' evaluations. However, it is possible that students may act differently in a simulated context or that simulated patients may give higher ratings to students who can 'play the game' in a high stakes examination setting (Berg et al. 2011). It may be that a person's beliefs in the importance of empathy are reflected in their practice. The reported decline in student empathy occurred at the same stage in the students' education, when they entered the clinical years (Hojat et al. 2009).

The JSPE is based on an assumption that cognition is of a higher order than emotional aspects of care thus ignoring the social and cultural research showing the interconnection between cognition and emotion (Hooker 2015; Kozlowski et al. 2017). Most of the JSPE questionnaire items surveyed students' attitudes towards empathy and related phenomena rather than empathy in practice. Furthermore, the JSPE did not distinguish between empathy, compassion, active listening or other forms of engaged clinical care. Hooker (2015) argued that the JPSE tells us little that is meaningful about empathy but more about how the medical profession perpetuates myths about an emotionally invulnerable doctor (Hooker 2015). Other authors have concluded that the self-reported instruments used to record empathy may not be measuring anything meaningful (Sulzer et al. 2016; Pedersen 2009; Roff 2015). I concur with their view and would suggest that the JSPE questionnaire, with its emphasis on cognitive aspects, is of little relevance to the clinical context. Indeed, I suggest most of the quantitative measures can be similarly critiqued. One may legitimately ask: 'what exactly is the JPSE measuring? Is it a level, trait, capacity, resonance, skill or attitude?' (Hooker 2015).

The Conflicting Evidence for an Empathy Decline

An early quantitative study, using the JSPE, concluded that empathy declined in medical school (Hojat et al. 2004). This led to a concern reflected in journal article titles, such as 'Is there a hardening of the heart in medical school?', and an editorial entitled 'Decline in empathy in medical education; how can we stop the rot?' (Newton et al. 2008; Spencer 2004).

In a longitudinal study in the USA, 456 JSPE self-assessments were completed five times over the duration of the course with the authors finding that there was a decline in empathy scores at the end of the third year, which continued to graduation (Hojat et al. 2009).

Research in other countries also reported a decline in medical students' empathy during their training (Newton et al. 2008; Chen et al. 2007; Kliszcz et al. 1998; Lim et al. 2013; Shashikumar et al. 2014; Shariat and Habibi 2013; Austin et al. 2007; Youssef et al. 2014; Thomas et al. 2007; DiLalla et al. 2004; Stratton et al. 2008). Additionally, two systematic reviews of empathy in medical students concluded that empathy declined (Pedersen 2010; Neumann et al. 2011). Konrath et al. (2010) surveyed American college students, concluding that an empathy decline had become a social phenomenon in young Americans.

In a review of studies reporting an empathy decline in medical students, Neumann identified a number of methodological problems including low response rates, few longitudinal studies and a lack of information on gender and speciality (Neumann et al. 2011). Furthermore, few of these studies gave details of the medical curriculum or the context of the research (Quince et al. 2016a, b).

Roff (2015), however, disputed the reported decline in empathy. She pointed out that the evidence of an empathy decline in medical students was mainly based on research in the USA (Roff 2015). Roff (2015) reviewed studies from a dozen countries outside the USA, which in contrast showed a trend towards an increase rather than a decline in empathy, with the exception of studies by Shashikumar et al. (2014), from India, and Shariat and Habibi (2013), from Iran. A number of quantitative studies have reported either no change or an increase in empathy in medical students during their training (Hong et al. 2012; Mahoney et al. 2016; Magalhaes et al. 2011; Tavakol et al. 2011; Rahimi-Madiseh et al. 2010; Mostafa et al. 2014; Bratek et al. 2015; Kataoka et al. 2009; Roh et al. 2010; Costa et al. 2013). A scoping review of 209 international quantitative studies concluded that there was no generalised international trend in changes in student empathy throughout medical school (Ferreira-Valente et al. 2016).

Colliver et al. (2010), in their review of eleven studies, questioned the reported decline in medical students' empathy. They re-examined the results by transforming them back to their original rating scales and then examined the relationship between the empathy ratings and response rates (Colliver et al. 2010). They discovered that there was only a very small decline in mean ratings which, due to the low and varying response rates, was of doubtful significance (Colliver et al. 2010).

In the UK, Quince et al. (2011) carried out a longitudinal study of Cambridge medical students between 2007 and 2010, using a self-reported annual questionnaire which distinguished between affective and cognitive empathy (Quince et al. 2011). They found that neither men nor women appear to become less empathetic during medical education at Cambridge (Quince et al. 2011). Quince et al. (2016b) followed this study with a multi-centre (15 UK and 2 international medical schools), cross-sectional comparison of students at the start of their course and as they approached the end of their training, using an online questionnaire survey. The authors concluded that there was no evidence of an empathy decline but that questions remained concerning the trajectory of changes in empathy during medical student training (Quince et al. 2016b). This was supported by an Australian study that concluded:

> a more sophisticated understanding of empathy in medical students is needed, with attention to issues that might adversely impact on this crucial aspect of their development. (Mahoney et al. 2016, p. 270)

A striking finding in my research was that students described their empathy as developing rather than declining, especially after contact with patients. This finding is in marked contrast to the reports from quantitative studies of students' empathy declining in the clinical years of the course (Newton et al. 2008; Chen et al. 2007; Hojat et al. 2009). My research findings concurred with the quantitative research which reported either no change or an increase in empathy in medical students during their training (Magalhaes et al. 2011; Mahoney et al. 2016; Quince et al. 2011, 2016b). Although it was significant that students in my study claimed that their empathy had not declined but had actually increased, phenomenological research is concerned more with understanding their rich nuanced descriptions rather than quantifying the changes experienced by the students.

Millennial learners are said to demonstrate a tendency to narcissism, but these students told a different story, of an increasing interest in the other person (Twenge 2013). American surveys of preclinical medical students concluded that there was a loss of idealism during their training (Morley et al. 2013; Mader et al. 2014). However, in my study the students claimed the reverse was true, and they were becoming more sensitive to patients' needs, were enthusiastic about becoming doctors and wanted to include psychosocial aspects in their work.

A cross-sectional study, with a group of seven students in years 3 and 4 in a UK university, also showed some of these changes in students' empathy (Tavakol et al. 2012). The students in the phenomenological study carried out by Tavakol et al. (2012) regarded empathy as a personality trait rather than in a relational way. Some students described that their empathy had not declined, but their high clinical workload resulted in less overt demonstrations of empathy while others felt, like most of the students in my study, that their empathy had increased with patient contact (Tavakol et al. 2012). Their findings concurred with the views of some students in my research who identified a tension between empathy and efficiency, a tension described in other qualitative studies (Allen et al. 2008; Eikeland et al. 2014).

Students in my study gave a wealth of examples relating to greater sensitivity with patients despite their perceived barriers to empathy in the curriculum. They described how they had developed a more 'practical' form of empathy which involved appreciating the patient's emotions but at the same time focusing on the immediate medical problem. Their stories revealed a greater self-awareness of their relationship with patients. The relevance of the psychosocial lectures delivered in the first year was appreciated when students reached the clinical years.

The students described how initially they were self-conscious and nervous when talking to patients. Also, in early years, they described 'hunting for signs' in 'interesting' patients on the ward. Other studies have noted that some students regarded patients as cases, or learning resources, rather than people, which they suggested was one of the factors accounting for an empathy decline (Tavakol et al. 2012; Allen et al. 2008; Christakis and Feudtner 1997). However, in my study students described how their relationship with patients deepened in a process some described as 'getting it'.

Students acknowledged that the context of their encounter affected the level of empathy which they displayed, rather than how they felt emotionally. This tension between their empathetic attitude and more distanced behaviour when constrained by time reflects one of the many problems in assessing empathy (Rees and Knight 2007). Conrad (1988) proposed that in medical schools which emphasised technical aspects of medicine rather than caring, students struggled to maintain a humanistic perspective. He claimed that towards the end of their training some students shifted their perspective to become doctor-orientated rather than patient-orientated, a claim refuted by my research (Conrad 1988). It may be that students in my study were more humanistic in their outlook than some of their peers, but all of them described a shift in perspective from being student-orientated to patient-orientated.

The Preclinical Group: Finding 'a Doctor's Voice'

Students recalled their apprehension about their first contact with patients. Initially, they considered that some patients were uncommunicative, but they found it was because they were unable to empathise with them. At first, Helen considered empathy as a performance, describing how she felt as though she was pretending to be a doctor, as she gained in confidence she found her 'doctor's voice'.

> every time I put my stethoscope on I felt like a kid playing dress up. (Helen, Year 3)
>
> I think at the start I was so not nervous but flustered and not sure. Actually patients don't want to open up to you if you are a bit unsure of what you are asking and why you are asking and they don't feel like they can trust you. (Helen, Year 3)
>
> you find, your almost, a doctor voice. (Helen, Year 3)

Some students felt they were playing a role as 'doctor', resonating with descriptions of surface acting, in which the student appears empathetic but does not share any emotion with the patient (Larson and Yao 2005). Students described competence as creating a space for empathy; others called this process 'finding a doctor's voice' (Rosenfield and Jones 2004). Another study also found that in striving to accumulate factual knowledge students lost sight of the psychological aspects of care (Haas and Shaffir 1977). Although students in my study described instances where they seemed less emotionally connected to patients, they reflected on these experiences and adjusted their behaviour. They retained their motivation to have a close empathetic relationship with patients.

The preclinical group of students talked about the transitions they experienced from school to university. Some described this as a process of maturing, but others felt that they were being 'moulded' by the medical school to become a certain type of doctor.

> [pause] I don't think mature is the right word [laughing] [...] It is almost rather than you are maturing by yourself, you are being guided onto a path. So it is a weird thing, I have matured but almost I don't feel it is always an independent thing. (Bill, Year 3)

Connie compared this process to child development and described how she became more aware of the influence of context on empathy and the need to focus on the other person rather than herself. She implied that although it might appear from her behaviour that she had become more distant from patients at times, she still experienced the same emotions and felt empathy with patients.

> Professionalism isn't the opposite of empathy, but imagine it in the same way as a child growing up. A child will cry at anything and everything when it is not their way or sad or whatever. Whereas when you mature and become an adult you learn that sometimes you can't just make a situation about you, that you need to feel and understand what other people are going through and that the way you conduct yourself needs to change. (Connie, Year 3)

Students differentiated between developing resilience or as they described it, as being 'harder', while at the same time developing empathy, by being warmer with patients. Some also agreed that they may have become more cynical about certain issues, for instance the medical school's responsiveness to change or their increasing workload. However, they claimed that this form of cynicism did not affect their empathy with patients. In a Scandinavian study, some students described cynicism as an accepted coping strategy (Eikeland et al. 2014). My findings contrasted particularly with the early studies of professional socialisation which reported a development of cynicism (Becker and Geer 1958; Merton et al. 1957). In view of these different findings, there is now a need for further qualitative social science research into the process of professional socialisation.

A study of medical students' views on professionalism had parallels with the findings in my study (Monrouxe et al. 2011). In both studies, students had differing understandings of the phenomena, empathy and professionalism. Students who had delayed contact with patients had a restricted view of professionalism focused on dressing and acting as a professional (Monrouxe et al. 2011). However, those who experienced early patient contact developed a more sophisticated concept of professionalism (Monrouxe et al. 2011). The authors concluded that becoming a professional was an interpersonal and complex activity which needed to be nurtured in the formal curriculum (Monrouxe et al. 2011). These findings mirror those in my thesis in relation to empathy.

Edward described how his empathy had become both more refined and medicalised. He talked about differentiating between patients and people. He claimed that this did not mean he was less empathetic but acknowledged that when short of time, others might imagine he lacked empathy.

> I think my empathy is probably more refined than it was. I have more if an idea how an interaction to go and I tend to think of patients as patients, than just people you can meet in the street that happened be in front of you. (Edward, Year 4)

> My feelings towards people who come in as patients haven't really changed but I think outwardly if you were to watch me interact with patients I am probably less likely to jump in and go the personal stuff. I will still do it but it would have to be in right context. (Edward, Year 4)

Fiona considered that her attitude to empathy might have developed gradually throughout the course. She reflected that with increasing clinical competence she might have more space for empathy.

> I don't think differently but [...]if there was it would be a gradual thing which I wouldn't be able to lay a finger on. (Fiona, Year 3)

Connie described her empathy as being 'buried' during the early years of the course, but she now felt more confident making her empathy apparent.

> at least it is not as buried down, it comes to the surface a lot more. (Connie, Year 3)

Students claimed that they were more sensitive to patients' needs as they progressed through the course. This contrasted with early findings of students becoming more detached to retain objectivity (Coombs and Powers 1975). An American study found that students demonstrated a number of strategies for coping with emotions including objectifying the patient, accentuating the comfortable feelings that come from 'real medicine', blaming patients, humour and distancing (Smith III and Kleinman 1989). It has been argued that medical school education is a process of assimilation into a culture of objectivity (Gordon 1995).

Olive compared the difference between being resilient yet empathetic, or maintaining a cold, distant approach to patients. She claimed that resilience need not result in being colder towards patients. She claimed that 'colder' implied a loss of empathy but in fact she felt that her empathy had increased with more patient contact.

> you can be harder but don't need to be colder. I think you can [be] harder more you are resilient, you are more able to deal with these things. You don't get knocked back by every challenge. (Olive, Year 3)

> colder would be the lack of empathy, the lack of care, the lack of compassion. I would hope that as people progress through their medical career they become harder and more resilient. I would hope that as people see more patients and have greater understanding of what it means to be a patient and what different experience they have had they can be warmer. (Olive, Year 3)

Olive noticed that for some students the focus had changed from themselves to the patient, a process she described as 'getting it', though this realisation might not be achieved until the clinical years of the course.

> for some people it always been a lot more about the patient, 'I am really interested in learning about this because I know it is actually going to help me be a good doctor. I am not that bothered [...] because I might get an extra few marks it doesn't seem that important', and some people would be able to say that very very clearly, and whereas for others, it still at this stage about stuffing facts into your brain. (Olive, Year 3)

Haas and Shaffir (1977) proposed that changes in medical students began with the admission process when applicants adapted themselves to fit the perceived requirements of the university. Using data from participant observation and interviews, they found that faced with inordinate demands to display competence, students reacted by distancing themselves from patients, by adopting a 'cloak of competence' (Haas and Shaffir 1977). The authors argued that the symbols of the profession also separated them from patients (Haas and Shaffir 1977).

It was however, in the clinical years, that students described the most changes in their empathy.

The Clinical Group: The Patient–Student Relationship

Students in the latter years of the course felt greater confidence and increased empathy with their contact with patients. Their stories illustrated differing facets of their perceived changes in empathy as they reflected on their progress through their course and looked forward to working as doctors.

Kim said that she was fairly confident about her clinical competence and so felt less vulnerable. She suggested that this was partly due to having less factual material to learn. She contrasted her learning process in lectures where facts were 'thrown at you' with working on the wards where she 'picked things up' and understood the meaning of the new information.

> I suppose in a way I feel less vulnerable [...] I felt that I knew it less when we were in the lectures because the so much being thrown at you at once. Whereas especially when you have had a week or so on the wards you are starting to pick things up and take things in. (Kim, Year 4)

Kim, with increased self-awareness, reflected on her empathy when she attended a care course. She realised how 'medicalised' she had become as she tended to plunge in and ask patients direct intimate questions. She recognised that there was an appropriate time for direct questions and that it was not always the best approach.

> it was massive wake-up call and exactly how medicalised you become after two years of medical school and 6 months on the ward. (Kim, Year 4)

> I think because you are so used you going in and saying, you got a lanyard around your neck that says third year medical student on it, and you can go in and say to somebody, 'Tell me about your bowel habits today'. (Kim, Year 4)

Kim realised that she was causing embarrassment by asking intimate questions too early in the consultation. However, she reflected that while she might find such questioning straightforward, the patient might take a different view.

> one of the things about empathy is that immunity that you gain as you go through. [...] when you are going through medical training you are told to ask about bowel habits, you think this isn't going to be very easy [...] when they are telling you just go in and ask about it. You are thinking, 'Oh God I couldn't, I don't know if I will ever be able to do that'. (Kim, Year 4)

She described how clinical experience with patients deepened her empathy, but she still found it emotionally challenging. She appreciated the need to spend time with patients to establish empathy and described how taking a history enabled her to see a bigger picture.

> I think sometimes it has not diminished in that I still find myself getting quite I find it difficult let go of things sometimes. And I still find it very emotionally challenging in certain aspects. (Kim, Year 5)

She was aware that some people suggested that medical students became more cynical through their training, but she was unsure whether this was true. She talked about the ways she had developed her empathy by remembering each patient was an individual with differing needs.

> people say you become more cynical and I think in some ways that maybe is true. Um but then I don't know. (Kim, Year 6)

> you have got to remember for each family that is not normal, that is new, that is quite challenging. (Kim, Year 6)

Ida found that she now did not feel so overwhelmed when working with patients as she had been at the start of the course. However, she implied that there might be a risk of losing affective empathy in developing her resilience. Ida described how in gaining confidence she had become more empathetic and therefore ready to explore the patient's concerns. She reflected that she no longer saw patients simply as teaching resources.

> I am definitely more confident about more in the way that I am now quite happy to give out control of the chat [...]I am quite happy to let patients to take up a bit more control. And think they appreciate that they like it better. (Ida, Year 5)

> some of us would go to the wards and say 'are there any interesting patients'? Some doctors have said 'every patient is interesting'. (Ida, Year 6)

Amy described how she became disillusioned with medicine due to the scientific bias of the first years. However, she flourished in the clinical years as her empathy with patients developed. She felt she had a greater commitment to patients, a trend she shared with other students.

> in the clinical years when you get to see patients and how this problem affects them and affects their life and why you need to treat these problem it become more colourful. (Amy, Year 5)

> I think priorities have shifted since first year. Definitely people are more keen to get involved in things related to medicine. (Amy, Year 5)

Amy said that she had become more practical and gave an example of admitting a patient with anorexia nervosa who was acutely unwell. She reflected that in the early years she might have spent a long time exploring the patient's psychological issues but, in the final year, she realised that attending to the urgent medical problem was her priority.

> I didn't dwell [on] 'how is the mood?' I mean I did ask but quite quickly I suppose and tried to be empathic in my approach but it would not have been but perhaps two years ago I would have sat down really interested in

> her history […] I just tried to be more practical and efficient about it, to treat medical problems. (Amy, Year 6)

She was now more confident working in a team and talking to patients and said that in the final year she had a feeling that things were coming together.

> a few years ago in the clinical environment in year four we were trying not to step on toes and try to be hidden away in a sense. But now I think I am more comfortable working in a team, I am more comfortable talking to patients. (Amy, Year 6)

Lisa also claimed that her empathy improved during the clinical years. Prior to this, she was focused on the disease rather than the person. However, she qualified her claim by hinting that empathy was still an extra to the main medical agenda.

> Whereas now having nine months of meeting patients it is gotten better. Maybe my confidence has grown more so I feel I can venture into more empathetic area rather than doing what I am there for really. (Lisa, Year 4)

Lisa described seeing the patient as a person rather than a learning tool and having more confidence to explore the patient's ideas. She suggested that her increased confidence had created more space for empathy with the patient.

> I think now we are much more involved with patients and things so maybe seeing them in the beginning and getting to know them a bit more. And I think the more you know someone the more you can have empathy for them. (Lisa, Year 6)

> A lot more than seeing patients as learning tools rather than the patient as a person. (Lisa, Year 6)

Paula found that experience on the wards in meeting patients had helped develop her empathy. She remembered how nervous she was at the outset of the course. She described her increased confidence with patients and also of relating more closely to her colleagues in a process of professional socialisation.

> I was nervous about starting them because the first two years are 'sciencey' [...] This year it become second nature to be on the ward and talk to patients. (Paula, Year 4)

> I have gained a lot of confidence in terms of being able to approach a patient and speak to them and continue the conversation not worrying about that at all in the same way I would have been at the start. (Paula, Year 6)

> I now also relate better to other medics who are at the same stage as me we can appreciate what we doing is quite intense and seeing lot of real life, which I struggle sometimes to explain to people outside of medicine. (Paula, Year 6)

Paula commented that most of the change in empathy occurred in the clinical years and reflected how she had learned to control her emotions.

> On oncology I thought it was quite a heavy few weeks because of the kind of things you were seeing and I thought that is quite tough going through that which might suggest that there is empathy there that I was processing what I was seeing. (Paula, Year 5)

A recent experience with a patient who died made her wonder whether she had become a bit hardened to the situation. However, she suggested that her lack of emotion on this occasion might have been because she did not know the patient.

> I was surprised that I didn't feel more upset by it then I did. And I still don't really know why that is the case. I think it is probably there is an element of self-defence you can't get upset every time you see something like that, and also I didn't know that patient. (Paula, Year 6)

Paula implied that although she still felt empathy, the pressure for efficiency affected her relationship with the patient. She thought that the need to present the patient's problem to the consultant in a concise manner might make her appear less empathetic.

> possibly being a little less empathic when I think about the volume of patients I might have been sent to see. (Paula, Year 6)

> I see the patients myself and the goal of being able to present and exam back to someone and then do something about it. [...] I don't think that I am not empathetic with them because of that but I think it does maybe slightly change the way I will relate to them. (Paula, Year 6)

Gina suggested that her empathy had developed with maturity and described a shift to a greater commitment to patients. She now appreciated the relevance of the psychosocial lectures in first year.

> I think as you get more clinical experience you because a lot of what we did in first and second year was about the consultation process and social psychosocial model or whatever and appreciate that illness has many dimensions for the patient and you should be appreciative of that and you should be able to empathise with a patient. (Gina, Year 5)

Gina claimed that her empathy had developed from maturing and from her own experience of illness rather than any specific influence of the course. However, she reflected that having more clinical responsibility and contact with patients had influenced her empathy.

> I think for me the fact just being older and becoming an adult and having to do adult things like living away from home and even the mundane tasks that you think about that is real life for the average person and then like I said being ill and stuff that has influenced me more than I have been taught or has been addressed on the course. (Gina, Year 4)

> A lot more getting involved and a bit more responsibility seeing patients. (Gina, Year 5)

While almost all the students claimed that their empathy had increased, Gina reflected that she might have become more cynical about some things but emphasised that did not mean she was hardened towards patients. She said that it would be easy to become cynical and tired by the workload, but not by the patients. She perceived a common feeling of disillusionment amongst her peers.

> I think there are a lot of things that I am more cynical about. But I don't think that means I am hardened. I was cynical about things because I don't want to become more hardened. I want to still remain capable of seeing human side and remembering everyone's perception is not my own so the way I see things isn't the way things are necessarily. (Gina, Year 6)

> it would be very easy to become disillusioned and cynical and I think a lot of my peers people have. I have been speaking to particularly fifth year [...] everyone was feeling quite disillusioned and worn out and I think it is easy to see how people can become sort of just fatigued by the volume of things. (Gina, Year 6)

Gina had developed an interest in the psychosocial aspect of medicine and reflected that her attitude to these issues had changed completely after contact with patients.

> I have become aware of all these other things, because I was smart I used to think I had to do something scientific, one of the medical specialties, because they were somehow superior and less to do with social sciences or community based approach which is complete nonsense. [...]now that is what I want to do. (Gina, Year 6)

Diana said that her empathy has increased and found encouragement and feedback helped to give her confidence. She reflected on how anxious she was about talking to patients for the first time and how much this has changed with experience.

> the thing that terrified me the most coming into first year of med school and sitting at the end of a sick old man at the end of their bed and try and work out what to do and what to say and now especially since gen med [general medicine] I found that so useful because I had to do that over and over on my own. (Diana, Year 6)

> I had really good tutors who held my hand for the first two days and then really pushed me after that and just said that is not good enough you need to make a plan [....] so now I feel that I have had the feedback to say that I am OK at it. (Diana, Year 6)

> as you go through medical school your exposure to distressing things and needing empathy and feeling things about stuff increases. (Diana, Year 6)

In the clinical years, she gained experience in other people's lives, patients from very different backgrounds. Diana was aware that she came from a privileged background and that this could be a disadvantage in empathising with people.

> for a lot of people they have grown up in a middle class background they have not had any exposure with people who struggle with money, who have grown up around drugs, around crime and things like that and understand how those people's lives work and function. (Diana, Year 6)

She said that her empathy had increased but was unsure how much was due to maturing rather than the medical course.

> I think the core is still there but it difficult to tease out what is just growing, being older 18 to 23 rather than what is medical training. (Diana, Year 6)

> certainly, [I] have changed, hopefully for the better. (Diana, Year 6)

Neville reflected on developing empathy as a lifelong process which depended on patient contact and evolved in the light of that experience. He sought to understand rather than making judgements. Neville implied that that empathy was part of life skills picked up outside the formal curriculum and discussed the transitions between adolescence and adulthood. Neville felt more competent with experience and concluded that his empathy has developed during the course.

> Everyone who applies to med school is yeah I know what empathy is, and until you actually interact with a patient and you see it yourself I don't think you fully understand. And it is a lifelong process you will continue to change your views of it […] as you meet patients or they say certain things, share their experiences and that will change your views of how you should interact with them. (Neville, Year 4)

> just more understanding, more understanding of the bigger picture. Because when you are naive about the situations I think it is easy to make those judgements and not take a step back. I think that comes with maturity that there are other reasons why people might be doing the things they are doing. (Neville, Year 4)

Neville's views had changed in that he now appreciated the importance of the psychosocial aspects of patient care and that there was more to medical practice than pure science. He described how he balanced efficiency and empathy and felt that his empathy has become refined.

> I came into medical school the view thinking that medicine was all about science, how wrong was I. [laughs] The science is a given but what makes a good doctor is much more than that. (Neville, Year 6)

> I feel at times I have been efficient but when the time is right it is also important to be that human being. (Neville, Year 6)

Neville now maintained that empathy could be taught and he suggested that incorporating the humanities could be useful for its development.

> there was first year students there and were told to read some history, some medical history in humanities this is all useless yadda yadda yadda. And maybe I would have said the same thing back then but now with the reflection of four or five years of medical school behind me, I enjoy that. (Neville, Year 6)

Neville summed up his empathy development and the major influences on his empathy: role-modelling, experience with patients and reading novels.

> I think if I had to sum up my change in medical school I think it is seeing role models, getting the experience and actually reading books and putting all that in makes such a difference. It is not just one thing which changes you it's a whole complement of different things that influences how you are as a human being.[…] I have been fortunate to actually been exposed to these things. It is tough for young people to see difficult issues or dealing with death but actually having going through it and reflect on it I think and I hope that it will put me in a better position to be a good doctor and look after people. (Neville, Year 6)

The students in my study wished to connect emotionally with the patient and, with greater self-confidence, to expose their own vulnerability. Students in the clinical years came to understand the place of psychosocial care in medicine. Some students noticed that their empathy had become more 'practical'. They claimed that although they might postpone a discussion of psychosocial issues in order to manage the medical problems, they retained their empathetic concern for the patient. All students stressed that they wanted to continue to develop their empathy, but expected that it might be threatened by their working conditions in the future, reflecting similar concerns expressed by students in another study (Nogueira-Martins et al. 2006).

Students described transitions during their undergraduate experience. Some described a process of maturing from school and assuming adult responsibilities, while other described a process of moulding by the medical school culture. These resembled the gradual transitions described by Perry in a study of college students (Perry 1968). Other students in my study seemed to have an epiphany described by some as 'getting it', or speaking with 'a doctor's voice', where they suddenly grasped what being a doctor involved, a process resembling 'doctrinal conversion' (Davies 2014). Some students described the development of empathy as a lifelong process which was influenced by many factors outside the medical curriculum including, for example, their own experience of illness. This view is supported by research suggesting that empathy developed in a bell-shaped curve through life with a peak in late middle-age (O'Brien et al. 2012).

Observational studies of professional socialisation, most of which were conducted many years ago in the USA, described how students adopted an increasingly detached professional image as they moved through medical school (Becker et al. 1961; Merton et al. 1957; Fox 1957). These studies demonstrated that the cultural environment of the medical school was critical to the professional socialisation of the students. They also showed that there was little attention paid to the character of the individual student (Montgomery 2006). Montgomery has argued that a culture of objectivity and detachment, described in these early studies, can combine with a neglect of the individual student to create an ethos of self-sacrifice (Montgomery 2006, p. 167).

A qualitative study in the USA that explored medical students encounters with cadavers and with living patients found that students learned that they should not talk about their emotions, especially not to the medical faculty (Smith III and Kleinman 1989). The study described students neglecting emotional issues, which led to the dehumanising of patients. Students adopted strategies for coping with their emotions including objectifying the patient, emphasising the satisfaction from practicing 'real medicine' and distancing themselves emotionally from patients (Smith III and Kleinman 1989). Gordon also argued that medical undergraduate education was a process of assimilation into a culture of objectivity which did not foster empathy with patients (Gordon 1995).

Smith III and Kleinman (1989) showed how the scientific approach can be used as a strategy to manage emotions, since the standard way of presenting a case history encouraged the student to think impersonally (Smith III and Kleinman 1989). Sinclair (2004) developed this view by arguing that evidence-based medicine (EBM) fostered the notion of presenting the history as a 'case', rather than as an individual patient's story (Sinclair 2004). It appeared that there was a tension in medicine between describing the scientific clinical condition and understanding the patient's lived experience (Good and Good 1989).

Since these early studies, there have been changes in medical undergraduate curricula, as a result of initiatives such as the GMC's publication, *Tomorrow's Doctors*, which have led to an outcome-based approach to undergraduate medical education (General Medical Council 2009). One consequence of these changes is that the professional socialisation of medical students is now more defined (Underman and Hirshfield 2016). There have also been demographic changes in the medical student population with more female students and a racially diverse student community (Underman and Hirshfield 2016). These developments have occurred against a background of changes in clinical practice such as EBM, increasing patient consumerism and a sophisticated technology which stresses a biomedical view of medical practice (Howick and Rees 2017; Montgomery 2006; Underman and Hirshfield 2016). In view of these curricular developments, there is now a need for further sociological studies to investigate professional socialisation in medical students (Underman and Hirshfield 2016). The question arises as to whether students are still being trained to adopt 'detached concern' as seemed to be the case in my research. My study was conducted in a UK medical school with an international reputation for scientific research. Authors have commented that in such medical schools students may struggle to maintain a humanistic perspective (Conrad 1988; Coulehan and Williams 2003).

Future Concerns

The students' accounts of changes to their empathy suggested that it had developed and evolved to adapt to differing clinical contexts. The students were also concerned not to lose empathy during their years as foundation doctors. Looking ahead Gina had some fears for her empathy when working as a Foundation Year 1 doctor (FY1). She was aware of the risk of losing empathy but said that her self-awareness might be a mechanism of preserving it.

> that it is a concern, seeing how intense working as a junior it can be, be easy to see how you can become a bit disenchanted with the system, and the work and got no time to do a million tasks, how easy it would be to just end up just going through the motions and not really thinking about things and ever stop and taking the time. I think yeah definitely that is a worry in the future. But it is something to keep myself aware of. (Gina, Year 4)

Paula expressed concerns about whether her judgement would be clouded by her feelings in the future.

> morally I think I would like to be empathetic to each patient that I meet but I feel that by being this career that may actually change. I think, I probably would find it very difficult to be taking on the feelings of an another person. If I did that with every patient I do think I would struggle to do my job with a clear head because you have a responsibility to do your job. (Paula, Year 4)

Many students expressed worries that their empathy might be limited by the pressure of time when working as a foundation doctor. They all had hopes that in the future they would spend time with patients.

> one privilege of medical school we have the time just to sit and chat but what I have seen is that the FY1 do try really hard to make sure to talk to patients. (Ida, Year 4)

Paula talked about the risks of becoming stressed in the future. But Lisa said that she was looking forward to her foundation years and working in a team who would provide mutual support.

> So I am anticipating it being stressful, [laugh] it will be. (Paula, Year 5)

> I am actually quite looking forward it. Probably more than a lot of people. I think a lot of people find it quite scary. I think I have had quite a bit of experience and I am not too worried about asking the nursing staff. (Lisa, Year 4)

The students' stories and concerns revealed the significance that they gave to empathy and their wish to preserve it in future although they were wary that difficult working environments in the future might threaten their expression of empathy.

Key Points

- Students described their empathy as developing rather than declining during their training.
- Students in the preclinical group viewed empathy as a personal attribute, but in the clinical years, they saw empathy as a relational construct.
- The preclinical student group linked their increased self-confidence and clinical competence with being more empathetic.
- Students became patient-orientated rather than self-orientated as they moved through their course.
- Students wanted to continue to foster empathetic relationships with patients in the future.

References

Allen, D., Wainwright, M., Mount, B., & Hutchinson, T. (2008). The wounding path to becoming healers: Medical students' apprenticeship experiences. *Medical Teacher, 30,* 260–264.

Alnoman, N. (2014). *Consultation and Relational Empathy (CARE) Measure in Medical Students* (PhD). University of Dundee.

Austin, E. J., Evans, P., Magnus, B., & O'Hanlon, K. (2007). A preliminary study of empathy, emotional intelligence and examination performance in MBChB students. *Medical Education, 41,* 684–689.

Becker, H. S., & Geer, B. (1958). The fate of idealism in medical school. *American Sociological Review, 23,* 50–56.

Becker, H., Geer, B., Hughes, E., & Strauss, A. (1961). *Boys in White: Student Culture in Medical School.* Chicago: University of Chicago Press.

Berg, K., Majdan, J. F., Berg, D., Veloski, J., & Hojat, M. (2011). A comparison of medical students' self-reported empathy with simulated patients' assessments of the students' empathy. *Medical Teacher, 33,* 388–391.

Bratek, A., Bulska, W., Bonk, M., Seweryn, M., & Krysta, K. (2015). Empathy among physicians, medical students and candidates. *Psychiatr Danub, 27,* 48–52.

Chen, D., Lew, R., Hershman, W., & Orlander, J. (2007). A cross-sectional measurement of medical student empathy. *Journal of General Internal Medicine, 22,* 1434–1438.

Chen, D. C. R., Pahilan, M. E., & Orlander, J. (2010). Comparing a self-administered measure of empathy with observed behavior among medical students. *Journal of General Internal Medicine, 25,* 200–202.

Christakis, D., & Feudtner, C. (1997). Temporary matters: The ethical consequences of transient social relationships in medical training. *JAMA, 278,* 739–743.

Colliver, J. A., Conlee, M., Verhulst, S. J., & Dorsey, J. K. (2010). Reports of the decline of empathy during medical education are greatly exaggerated: A re-examination of the research. *Academic Medicine, 85,* 588–593.

Conrad, P. (1988). Learning to doctor: Reflections on recent accounts of the medical school years. *Journal of Health and Social Behavior, 29,* 323–332.

Coombs, R., & Powers, P. S. (1975). Socialization for death: The physician's role. *Journal of Contemporary Ethnography, 4,* 250–271.

Costa, P., Magalhaes, E., & Costa, M. J. (2013). A latent growth model suggests that empathy of medical students does not decline over time. *Advances in Health Sciences Education, 18,* 509–522.
Coulehan, J., & Williams, P. (2003). Conflicting professional values in medical education. *Cambridge Quarterly of Healthcare Ethics, 12,* 7–20.
Davies, N. (2014). Empathic nursing: Going the extra mile. *Practice Nursing, 25,* 198–202.
Dilalla, L. F., Hull, S. K., & Dorsey, J. K. (2004). Effect of gender, age, and relevant course work on attitudes toward empathy, patient spirituality, and physician wellness. *Teaching and Learning in Medicine, 16,* 165–170.
Eikeland, H. L., Ornes, K., Finset, A., & Pedersen, R. (2014). The physician's role and empathy—A qualitative study of third year medical students. *BMC Medical Education, 14,* 165–173.
Ferreira-Valente, A., Monteiro, J. S., Barbosa, R., Salgueira, A., Costa, P., & Costa, M. J. (2016). Clarifying changes in student empathy throughout medical school: A scoping review. *Advances in Health Sciences Education, 22,* 1–21.
Fox, R. (1957). Training for uncertainty. In P. Merton, G. Reader, & P. Kendall (Eds.), *The Student Physician.* Cambridge, MA: Harvard University Press.
General Medical Council. (2009). *Tomorrow's Doctors: Outcomes and Standards for Undergraduate Medical Education.* London: General Medical Council.
Glaser, K. M., Markham, F. W., Adler, H. M., McManus, P., & Hojat, M. (2007). Relationships between scores on the Jefferson scale of physician empathy, patient perceptions of physician empathy, and humanistic approaches to patient care: A validity study. *Medical Science Monitor, 13,* 291–294.
Good, M. J. D., & Good, B. J. (1989). Disabling practitioners—Hazards of learning to be a doctor in American medical education. *American Journal of Orthopsychiatry, 59,* 303–309.
Gordon, L. (1995). Mental health of medical students: The culture of objectivity in medicine. *The Pharos of Alpha Omega Alpha-Honor Medical Society, 59,* 2–10.
Haas, J., & Shaffir, W. (1977). The professionalization of medical students: Developing competence and a cloak of competence. *Symbolic Interaction, 1,* 71–88.
Hemmerdinger, J. M., Stoddart, S. D. R., & Lilford, R. J. (2007). A systematic review of tests of empathy in medicine. *BMC Medical Education, 7,* 24.

Hojat, M., Mangione, S., Nasca, T. J., Cohen, M. J. M., Gonnella, J. S., Erdmann, J. B., et al. (2001). The Jefferson scale of physician empathy: Development and preliminary psychometric data. *Educational and Psychological Measurement, 61,* 349–365.

Hojat, M., Mangione, S., Nasca, T. J., Rattner, S., Erdmann, J. B., Gonnella, J. S., et al. (2004). An empirical study of decline in empathy in medical school. *Medical Education, 38,* 934–941.

Hojat, M., Vergare, M. J., Maxwell, K., Brainard, G., Herrine, S. K., Isenberg, G. A., et al. (2009). The devil is in the third year: A longitudinal study of erosion of empathy in medical school. *Academic Medicine, 84,* 1182–1191.

Hong, M., Lee, W. H., Park, J. H., Yoon, T. Y., Moon, D. S., Lee, S. M., et al. (2012). Changes of empathy in medical college and medical school students: 1-year follow up study. *BMC Medical Education, 12,* 122–127.

Hooker, C. (2015). Understanding empathy: Why phenomenology and hermeneutics can help medical education and practice. *Medicine, Health Care and Philosophy, 18,* 541–552.

Howick, J., & Rees, S. (2017). Overthrowing barriers to empathy in healthcare: Empathy in the age of the internet. *Journal of the Royal Society of Medicine, 110,* 1–6.

Howick, J., Steinkopf, L., Ulyte, A., Roberts, N., & Meissner, K. (2017). How empathic is your healthcare practitioner? A systematic review and meta-analysis of patient surveys. *BMC Medical Education, 17,* 136–145.

Kataoka, H., Koide, N., Ochi, K., Hojat, M., & Gonnella, J. S. (2009). Measurement of empathy among japanese medical students: Psychometrics and score differences by gender and level of medical education. *Academic Medicine, 84,* 1192–1197.

Kliszcz, J., Hebanowski, M., & Rembowski, J. (1998). Emotional and cognitive empathy in medical schools. *Academic Medicine, 73,* 541.

Konrath, S. H., O'Brien, E. H., & Hsing, C. (2010). Changes in dispositional empathy in American college students over time: A meta-analysis. *Personality and Social Psychology Review, 15,* 180–198.

Kozlowski, D., Hutchinson, M., Hurley, J., Rowley, J., & Sutherland, J. (2017). The role of emotion in clinical decision making: An integrative literature review. *BMC Medical Education, 17,* 255–268.

Larson, E., & Yao, X. (2005). Clinical empathy as emotional labor in the patient-physician relationship. *JAMA, 293,* 1100–1106.

Lim, B. T., Moriarty, H., Huthwaite, M., Gray, L., Pullon, S., & Gallagher, P. (2013). How well do medical students rate and communicate clinical empathy? *Medical Teacher, 35,* 946–951.

Mader, E. M., Roseamelia, C., & Morley, C. P. (2014). The temporal decline of idealism in two cohorts of medical students at one institution. *BMC Medical Education, 14,* 58–69.

Magalhaes, E., Salgueira, A. P., Costa, P., & Costa, M. J. (2011). Empathy in senior year and first year medical students: A cross-sectional study. *BMC Medical Education, 11,* 52–59.

Mahoney, S., Sladek, R., & Neild, T. (2016). A longitudinal study of empathy in pre-clinical and clinical medical students and clinical supervisors. *BMC Medical Education, 16,* 270–278.

Mercer, S. W., Maxwell, M., Heaney, D., & Watt, G. C. (2004). The consultation and relational empathy (CARE) measure: Development and preliminary validation and reliability of an empathy-based consultation process measure. *Family Practice, 21,* 699–705.

Mercer, S. W., McConnachie, A., Maxwell, M., Heaney, D., & Watt, G. (2005). Relevance and practical use of the consultation and relational empathy (CARE) measure in general practice. *Family Practice, 22,* 328–334.

Merton, R. K., Reader, G., & Kendall, P. L. (1957). *The Student Physician: Introductory Studies in the Sociology of Medical Education.* Cambridge, MA: Harvard University Press.

Monrouxe, L. V. (2010). Identity, identification and medical education: Why should we care? *Medical Education, 44,* 40–49.

Monrouxe, L. V., Rees, C. E., & Hu, W. (2011). Differences in medical students' explicit discourses of professionalism: Acting, representing, becoming. *Medical Education, 45,* 585–602.

Montgomery, K. (2006). *How Doctors Think: Clinical Judgment and the Practice of Medicine.* Oxford: Oxford University Press.

Morley, C. P., Roseamelia, C., Smith, J. A., & Villarreal, A. L. (2013). Decline of medical student idealism in the first and second year of medical school: A survey of pre-clinical medical students at one institution. *Medical Education Online* [Online], 18. Available https://doi.org/10.3402/meo.v18i0.21194. Accessed January 29, 2018.

Mostafa, A., Hoque, R., Mostafa, M., Rana, M. M., & Mostafa, F. (2014). Empathy in undergraduate medical students of Bangladesh: Psychometric analysis and differences by gender, academic year, and specialty preferences. *ISRN Psychiatry, 2014,* 1–8.

Neumann, M., Edelhaeuser, F., Tauschel, D., Fischer, M. R., Wirtz, M., Woopen, C., et al. (2011). Empathy decline and its reasons: A systematic review of studies with medical students and residents. *Academic Medicine, 86,* 996–1009.
Newton, B., Barber, L., Clardy, J., Cleveland, E., & O'Sullivan, P. (2008). Is there hardening of the heart during medical school? *Academic Medicine, 83,* 244–249.
Nogueira-Martins, M. C. F., Nogueira-Martins, L. A., & Turato, E. R. (2006). Medical students' perceptions of their learning about the doctor–patient relationship: A qualitative study. *Medical Education, 40,* 322–328.
O'Brien, E., Konrath, S. H., Grühn, D., & Hagen, A. L. (2012). Empathic concern and perspective taking: Linear and quadratic effects of age across the adult life span. *Journals of Gerontology Series B, 68,* 168–175.
Pedersen, R. (2009). Empirical research on empathy in medicine—A critical review. *Patient Education and Counseling, 76,* 307–322.
Pedersen, R. (2010). Empathy development in medical education—A critical review. *Medical Teacher, 32,* 593–600.
Perry, W. (1968). *Forms of Intellectual and Ethical Development in the College Years.* New York: Holt, Rinehart and Winston.
Price, S., Mercer, S., & Macpherson, H. (2006). Practitioner empathy, patient enablement and health outcomes: A prospective study of acupuncture patients. *Patient Education and Counseling, 63,* 239–245.
Quince, T. A., Parker, R. A., Wood, D., & Benson, J. A. (2011). Stability of empathy among undergraduate medical students: A longitudinal study at one UK medical school. *BMC Medical Education, 11,* 90–99.
Quince, T., Thiemann, P., Benson, J., & Hyde, S. (2016a). Undergraduate medical students' empathy: Current perspectives. *Advances in Medical Education and Practice, 7,* 443–455.
Quince, T. A., Kinnersley, P., Hales, J., da Silva, A., Moriarty, H., Thiemann, P., et al. (2016b). Empathy among undergraduate medical students: A multi-centre cross-sectional comparison of students beginning and approaching the end of their course. *BMC Medical Education, 16,* 92–102.
Rahimi-Madiseh, M., Tavakol, M., Dennick, R., & Nasiri, J. (2010). Empathy in Iranian medical students: A preliminary psychometric analysis and differences by gender and year of medical school. *Medical Teacher, 32,* 471–478.
Rees, C. E., & Knight, L. V. (2007). The trouble with assessing students' professionalism: Theoretical insights from sociocognitive psychology. *Academic Medicine, 82,* 46–50.

Roff, S. (2015). Reconsidering the "decline" of medical student empathy as reported in studies using the Jefferson scale of physician empathy-student version (JSPE-S). *Medical Teacher, 37,* 783–786.
Roh, M.-S., Hahm, B.-J., Lee, D. H., & Suh, D. H. (2010). Evaluation of empathy among Korean medical students: A cross-sectional study using the Korean version of the Jefferson scale of physician empathy. *Teaching and Learning in Medicine, 22,* 167–171.
Rosenfield, P. J., & Jones, L. (2004). Striking a balance: Training medical students to provide empathetic care. *Medical Education, 38,* 927–933.
Shariat, S. V., & Habibi, M. (2013). Empathy in Iranian medical students: Measurement model of the Jefferson scale of empathy. *Medical Teacher, 35,* 913–918.
Shashikumar, R., Chaudhary, R., Ryali, V., Bhat, P., Srivastava, K., Prakash, J., et al. (2014). Cross sectional assessment of empathy among undergraduates from a medical college. *Medical Journal Armed Forces India, 70,* 179–185.
Sinclair, S. (2004). Evidence-based medicine: A new ritual in medical teaching. *British Medical Bulletin, 69,* 179–196.
Smith III, A. C., & Kleinman, S. (1989). Managing emotions in medical school: Students' contacts with the living and the dead. *Social Psychology Quarterly*, 52, 56–69.
Spencer, J. (2004). Decline in empathy in medical education: How can we stop the rot? *Medical Education, 38,* 916–918.
Stratton, T. D., Saunders, J. A., & Elam, C. L. (2008). Changes in medical students' emotional intelligence: An exploratory study. *Teaching and Learning in Medicine, 20,* 279–284.
Sulzer, S. H., Feinstein, N. W., & Wendland, C. L. (2016). Assessing empathy development in medical education: A systematic review. *Medical Education, 50,* 300–310.
Tavakol, S., Dennick, R., & Tavakol, M. (2011). Empathy in UK medical students: Differences by gender, medical year and specialty interest. *Education for Primary Care, 22,* 297–303.
Tavakol, S., Dennick, R., & Tavakol, M. (2012). Medical students' understanding of empathy: A phenomenological study. *Medical Education, 46,* 306–316.
Thomas, M. R., Dyrbye, L. N., Huntington, J. L., Lawson, K., Novotny, P. J., Sloan, J. A., et al. (2007). How do distress and well-being relate to medical student empathy? A multicenter study. *Journal of General Internal Medicine, 22,* 177–183.

Twenge, J. M. (2013). The evidence for generation me and against generation we. *Emerging Adulthood, 1,* 11–16.

Underman, K., & Hirshfield, L. E. (2016). Detached concern?: Emotional socialization in twenty-first century medical education. *Social Science and Medicine, 160,* 94–101.

Youssef, F. F., Nunes, P., Sa, B., & Williams, S. (2014). An exploration of changes in cognitive and emotional empathy among medical students in the Caribbean. *International Journal of Medical Education, 5,* 185.

9

Summary and Implications

Overview

This chapter summarises the key findings of my research which I hope will resonate with medical educators. I hope that this book increases our understanding of the way in which students conceptualised empathy and highlights the factors in the curriculum which influenced their empathy. The overarching theme that emerged from the students' stories was the tension between emotional connection with and detachment from patients. The limitations of this phenomenological research are discussed. The contributions of this study to medical undergraduate education and to patient care are discussed. Although any conclusions drawn from a phenomenological study are necessarily tentative, the implications of my findings for research, education and practice are debated.

D. I. Jeffrey, *Exploring Empathy with Medical Students*,
https://doi.org/10.1007/978-3-030-11211-0_9

Summary of Findings

The study showed that initially, the students adopted an intrapersonal view of empathy, regarding it as an individual attribute. Later, with clinical experience, students took a different view of empathy, describing it as an interpersonal construct, which was dependent on the context of their contact with patients.

In exploring the relational concept of empathy, students described, in detail, the process of empathising with a patient. They reflected on establishing rapport, sharing emotions and the setting of an appropriate self-other boundary. They suggested that the different dimensions of empathy might combine flexibly to meet the needs of the individual patient. Some students described varying levels of empathy might be appropriate for differing clinical situations. They discussed how their empathy was affected by the context of their consultation with the patient.

The students rejected 'detached concern' as an appropriate model of medical professionalism. Instead, they expressed a wish to connect emotionally in empathising with patients. They described the benefits of empathy not only to patients, but also to themselves. Empathy generated a feeling of being valued and supported that led to their engagement and increased self-esteem. With such increased self-confidence, they felt able to open up to patients and were enabled to value others.

The research identified a range of factors which the students described as influencing their empathy. Their stories made explicit a variety of implicit influences in the hidden curriculum. Students described their clinical experience with real patients as the most significant positive influences on their empathy. The opportunity to develop a patient–student relationship was central to empathising and was enhanced by support from experienced clinicians. Such positive role models were clinicians who were willing to discuss emotional aspects of care, share their vulnerability and provide support to students. Students observed their clinical tutors' behaviour closely and described their impact on their own style of consultations with patients. The climate of the medical school exerted a profound influence; a relaxed positive learning environment fostered empathy development.

Students talked more about negative rather than positive influences during their training. They perceived barriers to empathy which distanced them from patients, primarily a conforming, competitive culture in the medical school in which they did not feel that they were valued as individuals. A more detailed analysis revealed other barriers to their empathy including a lack of patient contact, negative role models, a biomedical bias to their teaching and learning professionalism as 'detached concern' for patients. They suggested that their communication skills training with simulated patients encouraged a 'fake' empathy.

However, despite these negative influences in the curriculum, most students preferred to connect emotionally with patients. Some voiced concerns that sharing emotions might cause burnout or affect their objective clinical judgement. Others appreciated that sharing emotions might lead them to a fuller understanding of the patients' world, which would improve not only the care of the patient but also their job satisfaction. These students suggested that emotions should inform their clinical decision-making.

The students voiced a need for guidance on how to achieve an appropriate balance between connection and detachment in the student–patient relationship. They also expressed the need for support when they were engaging emotionally with patients. They identified consultations which both challenged and developed their empathy: talking to dying patients and to those with mental health problems. The students expressed a need for more guidance on empathising with people from differing ethnic backgrounds and cultures. Students stressed that they needed time to build an empathetic relationship. They identified a tension between empathy and efficiency in their clinical work. They also emphasised the negative effect of stress on their ability to empathise with patients.

Students maintained that they had developed their sensitivity to patients in the clinical years. However, they admitted to adopting behaviours, on occasions, to hide their empathy in the interests of efficiency, revealing the tension which existed between empathy and efficiency.

Empathy or Detached Concern?

The overarching theme identified by the students was the tension between connecting with patients emotionally, in relational empathy, and distancing themselves, by adopting 'detached concern'. At the heart of the medical undergraduate learning experience is the patient–student relationship. Students indicated that if this is to be an effective relationship, they needed to be encouraged to build an empathetic dialogue with patients. Students described a need for help in regulating their emotions: by distinguishing between appropriate empathetic concern and harmful personal distress; by creating an appropriate self-other boundary. Emotional engagement also depended on a learning environment which valued time spent with patients and which fostered continuity of care. They stressed that they wanted to have close relationships with patients but perceived that they had to act in a detached way in order to appear professional.

Limitations of the Research

Paley (2017, p. 17) criticised phenomenological qualitative research on the basis that 'bracketing' was impossible and that meaning-attribution problematic. In particular, he argued that a phenomenological analysis was simply a reflection of the researcher's own priorities (Paley 2017, p. 31). However, Paley in his criticism of phenomenology adopted a positivist stance, which was not theoretically consistent with a qualitative methodology (Paley 2017).

In Western society, the positivist ideas of science prevail to an extent that science is assumed to represent uninfluenced reality beyond interpretation (Montgomery 2006). Perhaps it is not surprising then that medicine distrusts anecdotes. Yet, paradoxically, clinical medicine begins with a patient's story. Phenomenological research and clinical medicine rely both on a negotiation, between the individual story and the background evidence, and on interpretation (Montgomery 2006).

One of the inevitable limitations of research in the social sciences is that it can never be possible to know fully what another person is thinking and feeling. However, the fact that a perfect understanding is not possible does not invalidate the knowledge generated by thorough, sensitive qualitative research (Finlay and Gough 2008). I have acknowledged, from my Heideggerian perspective, that it was not possible to remove all my assumptions about empathy. However, a phenomenological study demands reflexivity to make the researcher's position explicit. Paley seemed to ignore the fact that the aim of phenomenological qualitative research is to find meaning through the entire phenomenological research process, using interpretation and the relationship between the perceiver and the perceived (Sohn 2017).

My study was concerned with the students' experiences during their undergraduate education. Early influences on their empathy such as their upbringing and schooling, although potentially significant, were not investigated. The study was limited to a small number of a self-selected sample of students in one medical school in the UK. My method of recruiting students who volunteered for the study on a self-selected purposive basis was designed to recruit students who were motivated by the subject and were ready to commit to a study over three academic years. I anticipated that there would be attrition in the numbers of students volunteering for the research but found that they all attended every interview. The students who volunteered for the study were already engaged with the topic of empathy and so were probably not representative of all the students in the year group. Indeed, sometimes they sent e-mails to ask for an interview or to send interesting references. Their feedback indicated that participating in the study had increased their awareness of empathy. Rather than viewing their subjectivity as a bias, my theoretical approach and my research were enriched by their interest and commitment. My phenomenological research was concerned with exploring their subjective perspectives rather than achieving a representative sample.

There is scope to explore the relationship of gender, culture and power to the development of empathy, areas which were not considered in depth in my study. I suggest that further phenomenological studies are needed to deepen our understanding of the effects of these factors on empathy.

The study was limited to exploring the views of medical students and their experiences in the context of their medical education. It was beyond the remit of the study to consider the views of patients or the medical educators.

Quantitative studies were not included in this thesis as the phenomenological theoretical approach underpinning the study explores understanding rather than measurement of empathy. My phenomenological study was concerned with the medical students' everyday experiences; therefore, research in the neurosciences, describing neural pathways involved with empathising, was not discussed in my thesis but is described in *The Social Neuroscience of Empathy* (Decety and Ickes 2011). Integrating the neurosciences with social sciences is a new approach in research into empathy which has helped to validate, at a neurological level, the distinction between personal distress and empathetic concern (Decety and Ickes 2011).

Contribution to Education and Practice

The main contribution offered by my research is to increase understanding of the ways in which medical students perceive empathy and the factors which influence their empathy during their undergraduate training. By using an innovative method in medical education research, the study also contributes to research methodology.

The study responded to a need identified by many quantitative researchers for further qualitative research into the development of medical students' empathy. This is the first report in the literature of a longitudinal, phenomenological, interpretative approach to study empathy in medical students. It is also an innovative study, in its exploration of empathy, a construct which is integral to a phenomenological approach. This study has demonstrated how such an approach to data analysis can be used to gain new insights into the students' views and experiences of empathy.

The study contributed to a greater understanding of the complexity of empathy. It showed that students developed a relational view of empathy rather than viewing it as simply a personal attribute. This relational approach can be contrasted with the focus in the medical education literature which conceptualises empathy as a measurable personal attribute.

The study explored the process of empathising, highlighting key areas including rapport, sharing emotions, vulnerability and the self-other boundary. The students discussed how such an appropriate boundary might be formed and emphasised their need for guidance in this process from experienced clinicians.

The research demonstrated that the widely accepted belief that medical students lose empathy during their training concealed a more complex picture. They suggested that rather than losing empathy in the clinical curriculum, it developed as they focused on the student–patient relationship. However, on occasions they suggested it was necessary to hide their empathy.

The study revealed the impact of the context of the meeting between a patient and a student on the development of an empathetic relationship. In their stories, the students identified factors in the explicit and hidden curricula which influenced their empathy. Their insights may inform medical educators who wish to ensure that medical graduates are both competent and caring. The key factors from my research may be summarised as follows:

- The patient–student relationship

Students identified patient contact as the most influential factor in enhancing their empathy. Conversely, they described their lack of patient contact as inhibiting their empathy. Despite the rhetoric from the medical school concerning the desirability of patient-centred education, students identified missed opportunities to involve patients in their training. They further identified factors affecting their empathy including a decline in bedside teaching and a greater emphasis on simulation for both teaching and assessment of clinical skills.

- Role models

This research confirmed earlier findings which have shown how both positive and negative role models can influence students' empathy (Lempp and Seale 2004). Personal interaction is central to enhancing empathy. Positive role models are those teachers who relate to students as colleagues. They demonstrate in their work and teaching that the personal, emotional, moral and academic aspects of medicine are intertwined (Cooper 2011).

- Biomedical bias to teaching

The students identified a lack of teaching on empathy in the curriculum and limited guidance on managing their emotions or those of the patients. In the medical school, there appeared to be an increasing emphasis on biomedical science and a corresponding neglect of the psychosocial elements of care. Students described how the emphasis on the biomedical aspects of patient management contributed to an emotional distancing from patients.

- Professionalism as distancing from patients

The students perceived that their teaching on professionalism continued to be directed towards detachment from patients.

- The medical school culture

The research adds to our understanding of implicit factors that affect empathy in the hidden curriculum by making them explicit. These included the competitive environment, negative role models and a lack of psychological support or empathy for the students. There are other influences which affected the climate of the medical school, many of which lie outside the university, reflecting government policies and the interface between the university and the NHS. These aspects of medical education lie outside the scope of this study (Genn 2001). The values transmitted by clinical teachers to students in some ways may reflect how these educators feel valued by the university and NHS (Cooper 2011).

- Stress and support

Student support is essential for students to flourish and to enable them to be empathetic. Students show empathy when they feel positive and safe in the consultation (Cooper 2011). The study demonstrated that the students perceived support to be variable and dependent on the commitment of the personal tutor. The students were ambivalent about resilience, some describing it as incorporating empathy, while others argued that it implied detachment from patients.

It may appear that medical education research loses sight of its ultimate aim which is to improve patient care (Cleland 2015). The study contributed to practice by identifying elements of teaching which enhanced the students' empathy, and barriers which could inhibit it. The students acknowledged empathy as an essential part of being a good doctor. They identified their relationship with patients as being central to developing empathy and expressed their wish to be empathetic doctors. They hoped that their working conditions in the future would allow them to develop empathetic relationships with patients.

The students also identified clinical situations which both challenged and developed their empathy, for example in psychiatry and end-of-life care. They identified a potential tension between empathy and efficiency in clinical practice, highlighting the importance of time and continuity in developing empathetic relationships with patients.

Implications

In any phenomenological research, drawing implications must be tentative. Nevertheless, the following suggestions for the future are offered for debate.

The study demonstrated that interpretative phenomenological analysis (IPA), used in a longitudinal context, was a useful method for gaining an understanding of the students' world. My research suggested that the focus of future research in clinical empathy should explore empathy as a two-way relationship with the patient, rather than being an attribute of the student or doctor. It seems that rather than repeating quantitative measurements of empathy it would be more productive to carry out further longitudinal phenomenological research to explore the effects of the explicit and hidden curricula. There is a need to research the views of students in other medical schools, their medical educators and patients.

Implications for Medical Undergraduate Education

The implications for medical undergraduate education can be broadly described in two parts: changing the culture and introducing specific interventions to enhance empathy.

Culture Change

Medical undergraduate education is intimately linked to clinical care in the NHS. When situations arise such as the lapses in care described in the Francis Report, questions must be raised about the role and responsibility of medical education in creating the climate in which they occurred (Francis 2013). This research suggested that there needs to be a change in the culture of this medical school to remove the identified barriers to empathetic relationships between patients and students.

The study suggested that the medical school, which has an excellent reputation for biomedical research, needs to focus attention on psychosocial care. There is a need to give this subject the same value as the scientific elements of the curriculum. It is time for empathy to emerge from the hidden curriculum (Gallagher et al. 2017). Medical education, and clinical practice, needs to integrate both the science and humanity of patient care by allowing students to express empathy with patients. Patients value empathetic and humane doctors. To enhance the students' inherent empathy, explicit consideration needs to be given as to how empathy is influenced by their experiences of their training (Gallagher et al. 2017).

The study demonstrated that the medical school could do more to support and show the students that they are valued. We should not underestimate the need for an investment of time and support for students to enable them to care for themselves and for others (Cooper 2011). There is a need to address the contextual issues identified in my research and acknowledge the central role of patients in medical education (Halpern 2001; Shapiro 2012; Bleakley and Bligh 2008). Placing the patient–student relationship at the heart of medical undergraduate education and increasing the students' opportunities for contact with patients would help them with the process of emotional regulation. Students need time with mentors to provide feedback on difficult emotional issues arising in practice (Bleakley and Bligh 2008). Medical educators need to reflect on the reasons why students gained a perception of medical professionalism as distancing themselves from patients.

Some students in the study were pessimistic that the medical school would listen to their views or that any change would occur, a view reflected by some authors in the literature (Bloom 1989; Burks and Kobus 2012). Forty years ago, in a seminal paper advocating a biopsychosocial approach to medicine, Engel wrote,

> Nothing will change unless or until those who control resources have the wisdom to venture off the beaten path of exclusive reliance on biomedicine as the only approach to health care. (Engel 1977)

Antonovsky described a salutogenic approach focusing on well-being which addresses some of the mechanistic elements of the prevailing biomedical view in medicine (Antonovsky 1996). His model suggested that when encountering stress a person identifies and uses resources gained through their life experience. Antonovsky described this ability to have a healthy orientation as a sense of coherence (Antonovsky 1996). Empathy is integral to developing a sense of coherence since it depends on being connected to others and one's surroundings. Antonovsky's holistic approach to health rather than disease requires empathy to remind healthcare professionals of the human individual who has the disease.

I have shown how students are willing to empathise and to adopt a phenomenological approach to the patient. It is possible that by incorporating phenomenology into the medical education culture, students would be enabled to use their innate curiosity to empathise with patients and to explore with them the meaning of their illness. A philosophical foundation of phenomenology embraces openness and uncertainty, so fostering empathy. Such an approach accepts imperfection and by adopting patient-centred narrative approach allows students to connect more closely with patients (Shapiro 2008). A shared willingness to feel and convey empathy may result in a culture shift in medicine from detached concern to adopting a broad view of empathy as a dynamic relational process.

Specific Interventions to Enhance Empathy

Medical educators need to engage students with the goals of empathy, its centrality in providing patient-centred care and emphasising its relational aspects. Interventions to enhance empathy can be selected according to the needs of the students, for example in the early years giving students an opportunity to talk about their feelings of vulnerability and lack of competence (Plotkin and Shochet 2018). Efforts to improve the training of students to be more empathetic need to take account of the context of their clinical encounters with patients.

- Patient experience

A relational view of empathy has implications for the students' education; it prioritises the patient's experience as a source of learning. The students suggested ways in which patients could be more involved in their education. The simplest approach would be for students to have more contact with patients from the beginning of the course (Schweller et al. 2017). Psychosocial issues and empathy could then be addressed in the context of a relationship between the student and the patient with mentoring from an experienced doctor rather than in didactic teaching (Monrouxe et al. 2011). Other initiatives could include a greater emphasis on the patient experience during the lectures and patient involvement with problem-based learning which then becomes patient-based learning (Bleakley and Bligh 2008).

- Reflective practice

Students tended to restrict their understanding of reflection to written contributions in their portfolios. However, in their interviews they highlighted the central role of reflection in the process of empathising. This research suggests that students would appreciate an opportunity to reflect on their practice with experienced clinicians, especially when not being assessed. Some authors suggest that conversations about empathy should be specifically addressed in the first year of the course (Schweller et al. 2017).

- Guidance on setting boundaries

The students identified a need for guidance on how to balance their emotional connection with appropriate detachment. They wanted to learn how to maintain an appropriate self-other boundary and to develop deep collaborative working relationships with patients. Experienced practitioners can mentor students by providing time for them to discuss their difficulties.

- Removing barriers

The students described the ways in which their empathy was inhibited and these barriers require attention. For example, medical educators could incorporate emotional connection into medical professionalism and value students as colleagues. Good role models are inspirational but poor ones perpetuate a distancing form of practice (Bleakley and Bligh 2008). Vulnerability needs to be acknowledged to allow humane empathetic behaviours to flourish. Students need to be encouraged to give honest feedback on both good and bad practice. Humiliation and bullying should not be tolerated, not even in light-hearted banter. Students should feel that they can report these issues without affecting their academic progress.

- Providing support

The study has demonstrated that students described being less empathetic when stressed. They described the provision of personal support in the university as variable and gave reasons for their reluctance to seek such help. The implication for the medical school is that students need motivated personal tutors with a willingness to engage with them.

- Introducing the humanities into the curriculum

Students in this medical school had very little opportunity to engage with the medical humanities in the curriculum. Many authors have shown the potential for the humanities to promote empathy in medical students. There is scope for inclusion of this aspect in this curriculum (Batt-Rawden et al. 2013; Shapiro et al. 2006; Charon 2001).

If these suggestions resonate with the readers and local medical educators, the lessons from this research may also be shared with other medical schools and other healthcare professionals.

Implications for Clinical Practice

This research suggested approaches which may be adopted by medical schools to encourage students to be more empathetic with patients and their colleagues. However, an interpersonal view of empathy implied that the context of the relationship is also of importance. It is not enough to train students to be empathetic and then expect them to work sensitively in situations where they are stressed, lack time or receive little support. However, if psychosocial issues are given a higher priority, the empathy gap may be reduced (Francis 2013).

My research has demonstrated that clinical practice and phenomenology share characteristics, a willingness to try and see the world from the other person's point of view and a commitment to reflexivity. Thirty years ago, Schön (1987, p. 321) argued that there was a need to incorporate phenomenology into teaching and clinical practice, and other researchers have echoed his call (Van Manen 2016; Vagle 2010; Carel 2016; Montgomery 2006). I hope that this book, which describes the students' views, may contribute to achieving this aim.

Concluding Comment

The students' stories have been woven together to reveal new patterns of understanding of empathy. I have been privileged to listen to the stories of their experiences. I have learned much from the students who remained caring empathetic people throughout the research. I hope that my reporting of the students' stories does them justice and will contribute to curriculum changes which foster empathy. Engaging with phenomenology has taught me to listen, engage with the student and to reflect on their perspectives.

> there are no short cuts, there is no short way around this, and you need to sit down and see people. (Neville, Year 5)

References

Antonovsky, A. (1996). The salutogenic model as a theory to guide health promotion. *Health Promotion International, 11,* 11–18.

Batt-Rawden, S., Chisolm, M. S., Anton, B., & Flickinger, T. E. (2013). Teaching empathy to medical students: An updated, systematic review. *Academic Medicine, 88,* 1171–1177.

Bleakley, A., & Bligh, J. (2008). Students learning from patients: Let's get real in medical education. *Advances in Health Sciences Education, 13,* 89–107.

Bloom, S. (1989). The medical school as a social organization: The sources of resistance to change. *Medical Education, 23,* 228–241.

Burks, D. J., & Kobus, A. M. (2012). The legacy of altruism in health care: The promotion of empathy, prosociality and humanism. *Medical Education, 46,* 317–325.

Carel, H. (2016). *The Phenomenology of Illness*. Oxford: Oxford University Press.

Charon, R. (2001). Narrative medicine—A model for empathy, reflection, profession, and trust. *JAMA, 286,* 1897–1902.

Cleland, J. (2015). Exploring versus measuring: Considering the fundamental differences between qualitative and quantitative research. In J. Cleland & S. Durning (Eds.), *Researching Medical Education.* London: Wiley.

Cooper, B. (2011). *Empathy in Education: Engagement, Values and Achievement.* London: Bloomsbury Publishing.

Decety, J., & Ickes, W. (2011). *The Social Neuroscience of Empathy*. Cambridge: MIT Press.

Engel, G. L. (1977). The need of a new medical model: A challenge for biomedicine. *Science, 196,* 129–136.

Finlay, L., & Gough, B. (2008). *Reflexivity: A Practical Guide for Researchers in Health and Social Sciences*. Chichester: Wiley.

Francis, R. (2013). *Report of the Mid Staffordshire NHS Foundation Trust Public Inquiry: Executive Summary*. London: HMSO.

Gallagher, P., Moriarty, H., Huthwaite, M., & Lim, B. (2017). Challenging some assumptions about empathy. *The Clinical Teacher, 14,* 437–440.

Genn, J. (2001). AMEE Medical Education Guide No. 23 (Part 2): Curriculum, environment, climate, quality and change in medical education—A unifying perspective. *Medical Teacher, 23,* 445–454.

Halpern, J. (2001). *From Detached Concern to Empathy: Humanizing Medical Practice*. Oxford: Oxford University Press.

Lempp, H., & Seale, C. (2004). The hidden curriculum in undergraduate medical education: Qualitative study of medical students' perceptions of teaching. *British Medical Journal, 329,* 770–773.

Monrouxe, L. V., Rees, C. E., & Hu, W. (2011). Differences in medical students' explicit discourses of professionalism: Acting, representing, becoming. *Medical Education, 45,* 585–602.

Montgomery, K. (2006). *How Doctors Think: Clinical Judgment and the Practice of Medicine*. Oxford: Oxford University Press.

Paley, J. (2017). *Phenomenology as Qualitative Research: A Critical Analysis of Meaning Attribution*. London: Taylor & Francis.

Plotkin, J. B., & Shochet, R. (2018). Beyond words: What can help first year medical students practice effective empathic communication? *Patient Education and Counseling, 101,* 2005–2010.

Schön, D. A. (1987). *Educating the Reflective Practitioner: Toward a New Design for Teaching and Learning in the Professions*. San Francisco: Jossey-Bass.

Schweller, M., Ribeiro, D. L., Celeri, E. V., & de Carvalho-Filho, M. A. (2017). Nurturing virtues of the medical profession: Does it enhance medical students' empathy? *International Journal of Medical Education, 8,* 262.

Shapiro, J. (2008). Walking a mile in their patients' shoes: Empathy and othering in medical students' education. *Philosophy, Ethics, and Humanities in Medicine, 3,* 10–21.

Shapiro, J. (2012). The paradox of teaching empathy in medical students. In J. Decety (Ed.), *Empathy: From Bench to Bedside*. Cambridge: MIT Press.

Shapiro, J., Rucker, L., & Robitshek, D. (2006). Teaching the art of doctoring: An innovative medical student elective. *Medical Teacher, 28,* 30–35.

Sohn, B. K. (2017). Phenomenology as qualitative research: A critical analysis of meaning attribution. *Issues in Mental Health Nursing, 38,* 528–529.

Vagle, M. D. (2010). Re-framing Schön's call for a phenomenology of practice: A post-intentional approach. *Reflective Practice, 11,* 393–407.

Van Manen, M. (2016). *Researching Lived Experience: Human Science for an Action Sensitive Pedagogy*. London: Routledge.

Index

D. I. Jeffrey, *Exploring Empathy with Medical Students*,
https://doi.org/10.1007/978-3-030-11211-0

FSC
www.fsc.org
MIX
Papier | Fördert
gute Waldnutzung
FSC® C083411

Kolibri 360 GmbH
Ferdinand-Jühlke-Straße 7
99095 Erfurt, Deutschland
produktsicherheit@kolibri360.de